MASTERING ASANAS

A Complete Guide to Yoga Postures

Technique, Alignment & Teaching Cues
for Safe, Effective Practice

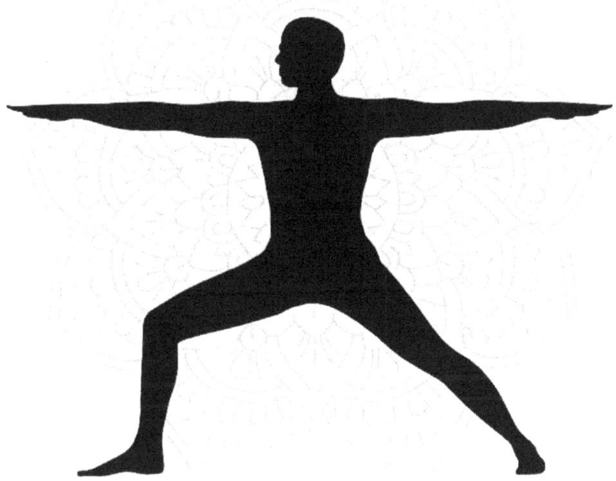

Published by:

YOGANTA

Yoga Alliance Registered School

Location: Hyderabad, India

Edition: May 2025

Website: www.yoganta.in

Email: hello@yoganta.in

YOGANTA

HEALTH | PEACE | HARMONY

Mastering Asanas: A Complete Guide to Yoga Postures

Compiled by Raushan Yoganta

First Edition – May 2025

ISBN: 978-93-343-0969-0

Published by Raushan Yoganta, Hyderabad, India

www.yoganta.in | hello@yoganta.in

TABLE OF CONTENTS

Introduction

Yoga postures—or asanas—are the most visible part of the yogic path, but their depth goes far beyond physical movement. An asana is not just a shape you create with your body—it is a state of presence, a bridge between breath, body, and awareness.

This book is designed to support both students and teachers in understanding and teaching asanas with clarity, intelligence, and respect for the body's natural structure. Whether you're deepening your own practice or preparing to guide others, you'll find detailed instructions, cues, and thoughtful insights into the art of mindful movement.

More than a list of poses, this guide teaches you how to see, feel, and share asanas with intention—focusing on function over form, awareness over aesthetics, and connection over perfection.

Let every posture be an invitation—not to perform, but to embody presence.

Wish You Health. Peace. Harmony

In gratitude,

Raushan Yoganta
Founder & CEO, Yoganta

Chapter 1: Introduction to Hatha Yoga

Hatha Yoga is one of the oldest and most foundational systems of yoga. It has evolved from ancient yogic texts like **Hatha Yoga Pradipika** by Swami Swatmarama, **Gheranda Samhita,** and **Shiva Samhita.**

The term '**Hatha**' is a combination of:

- "**Ha**" – meaning **Sun** (active, masculine, heating)
- "**Tha**" – meaning **Moon** (receptive, feminine, cooling)

Together, they represent the **balance of opposites** in the human body and experience.

Hatha Yoga is the practice of:

- **Physical postures (asanas)** to prepare the body
- **Breath control (pranayama)** to regulate life energy
- **Cleansing techniques (kriyas)** for purification
- **Inner awareness and stillness** for meditation

Yoga Asanas

"Asana" means **"seat"** or **"steady posture"** in Sanskrit. In classical yoga (as per **Patanjali's Yoga Sutras**), asana is described as:

"Sthira Sukham Asanam"

— A steady, comfortable posture.

Over time, the term expanded to include a variety of **physical postures** that prepare the body for **deeper yoga practice like meditation, breath control (pranayama), and spiritual evolution**.

Purpose of Asana in Yoga

- **Purifies and strengthens** the physical body
- **Balances energy** (Prana) through alignment of nadis (energy channels)
- Develops **discipline, focus, and self-awareness**
- Creates **stillness in movement** and builds the foundation for deeper yogic practices
- Prepares the body-mind for **meditation and inner awareness**

Chapter 2: Categories of Yoga Asanas

Asanas are often classified by their **physical orientation** and the effect they have on the body and mind. Grouping postures by category helps teachers plan balanced sequences, understand energetic impact, and offer appropriate modifications.

There are mainly **five categories** of asanas: **sitting**, **standing**, **supine** (lying on the back), **prone** (lying on the stomach), and **inverted**. Apart from these, there are also more specific categories like twists, forward bends, backward bends, balancing, core strengthening, restorative, etc.

1. Standing Asanas

- **Purpose**: Build strength, stability, balance, and grounded awareness.
- **Examples**: Tadasana, Trikonasana, Virabhadrasana I–III
- **Teaching Focus**: Foundation in feet, alignment through legs and hips, breath awareness.

2. Seated Asanas

- **Purpose**: Promote calm, focus, hip flexibility, and preparation for pranayama or meditation.
- **Examples**: Sukhasana, Padmasana, Baddha Konasana, Dandasana
- **Teaching Focus**: Neutral pelvis, lengthened spine, balanced grounding.

3. Supine Asanas (Lying on the back)

- **Purpose**: Relaxation, passive opening, core work, spinal mobility.
- **Examples**: Supta Baddha Konasana, Pavanamuktasana, Setu Bandhasana
- **Teaching Focus**: Pelvic alignment, supported breath, gentle spinal articulation.

4. Prone Asanas (Lying on the belly)

- **Purpose**: Strengthen the posterior chain, improve spinal extension, stimulate organs.
- **Examples**: Bhujangasana, Makarasana, Dhanurasana
- **Teaching Focus**: Core engagement, shoulder safety, compressive awareness.

5. Inverted Asanas

- **Purpose**: Reverse blood flow, stimulate nervous system, encourage introspection.
- **Examples**: Sarvangasana, Halasana, Viparita Karani
- **Teaching Focus**: Neck protection, smooth transitions, supported props when needed.

Principles of Alignment

Alignment in yoga is not about looking perfect—it's about **feeling connected, stable, and safe** within each posture. When the body is well-aligned, breath flows easily, effort is balanced, and injury risk decreases. Good alignment supports both the **physical and energetic intentions** of the pose.

Core Principles of Asana Alignment

Foundation First

Every pose begins at the base—whether it's the feet, hands, pelvis, or spine.

- Ground evenly through all contact points.
- Engage from the ground up to support upward lift or expansion.
- A strong foundation allows freedom in the rest of the body.

Neutral Spine & Pelvis Awareness

Understanding spinal curves and pelvic tilt is key in most asanas.

- Encourage a neutral spine unless intentionally flexing or extending.
- In standing and seated poses, align the pelvis to avoid strain.
- Tuck or untuck the tailbone based on pose demands—not as a rule.

Joint Stacking for Stability

Aligning joints vertically or in neutral planes reduces strain and builds strength.

- Example: In Tadasana, stack shoulders over hips, hips over knees, knees over ankles.
- Avoid hyperextension, especially in elbows and knees.
- Create "microbends" when needed for support.

Breath as an Alignment Tool

Breath reveals misalignment or tension.

- Smooth, steady breath = balanced alignment.
- If breath is strained, ease off, adjust, or support the pose.

Balance Effort and Ease (Sthira-Sukha)

- Sthira = steadiness, strength, active engagement
- Sukha = comfort, ease, relaxation
- In each pose, find the place between holding too tightly and collapsing.

Adaptation over Imitation

There's no one-size-fits-all in alignment.

- Teach to function, not just form.
- Respect each student's range of motion, body type, and experience.
- Use props or variations to meet the individual—never force alignment into pain.

Chapter 3: Pose Library

Sitting, Standing, Supine, Prone & Inverted

Sitting Yoga Asanas

DANDASANA - Staff Pose

Sanskrit Name: Dandasana - दण्डासन

English Name: Staff Pose

Category of Pose: Seated / Foundational

Level of Difficulty: Beginner

Step-by-Step Instructions:

- Sit on the mat with legs extended straight in front of you.
- Keep the feet together, toes pointing up.
- Press the thighs and calves gently into the floor.
- Place palms beside the hips, fingers pointing forward, arms straight.
- Engage the core and lift through the spine, keeping the back tall.
- Relax the shoulders away from the ears.

Benefits:

- Strengthens back muscles and improves posture.
- Activates hip flexors and core stability.
- Stretches shoulders and chest gently.
- Serves as a base posture for many seated forward bends.

Contraindications:

- Wrist or lower back injury - use props or modifications.
- Tight hamstrings - bend the knees slightly if needed.

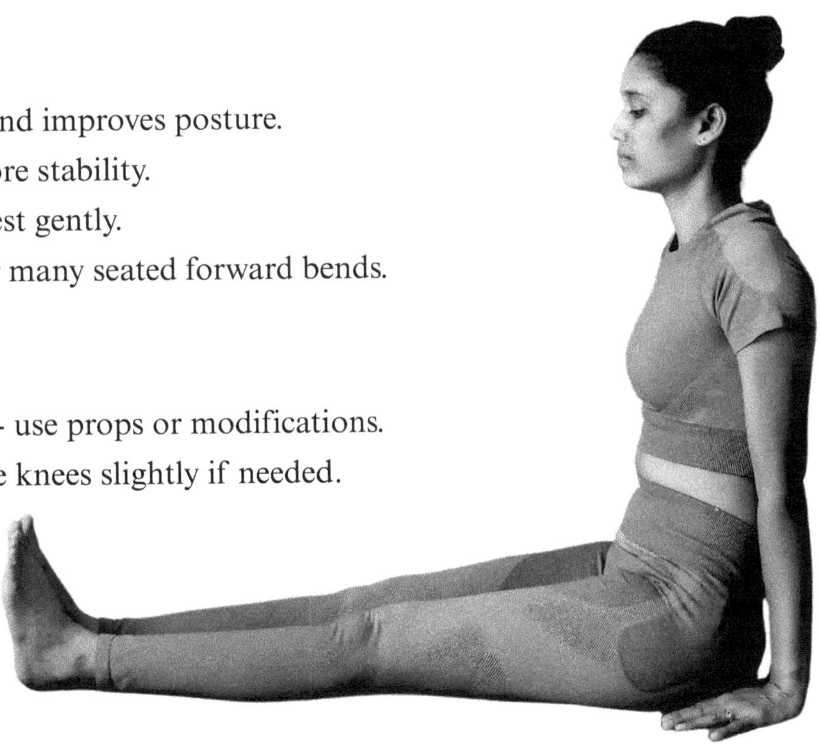

Dandasana

SUKHASANA – Easy Pose

Sanskrit Name: Sukhasana - सुखासन

English Name: Easy Seated Pose

Category of Pose: Seated / Meditative

Level of Difficulty: Beginner

Step-by-Step Instructions:

- Sit with legs extended forward (Dandasana).
- Cross the legs at the shins, letting knees fall outward.
- Sit evenly on both sit bones. Use a folded blanket if your hips are tight.
- Keep the spine upright and shoulders relaxed.
- Rest hands on knees or thighs, palms up or down.
- Close eyes or gaze softly forward. Breathe naturally.

Benefits:

- Gently opens hips and stretches knees and ankles.
- Encourages upright posture and spinal alignment.
- Calms the mind; excellent for breathwork and meditation.
- Grounds energy and promotes mental clarity.

Contraindications:

- Hip or knee injuries (use support or alternative seated pose).
- Sciatic pain (elevate hips to avoid strain).

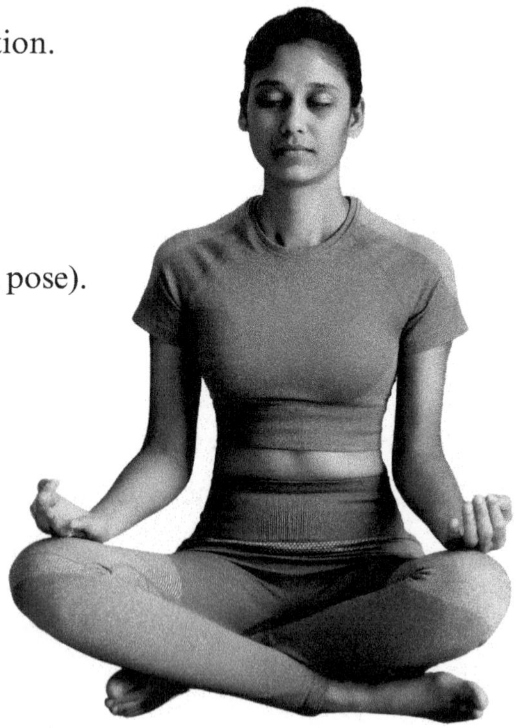

Sukhasana

Modifications & Props:

- Sit on a cushion or folded blanket to lift hips.
- Place yoga blocks or cushions under the knees for support.

PADMASANA - Lotus Pose

Sanskrit Name: Padmasana – पद्मासन

English Name: Lotus Pose

Category of Pose: Seated / Meditative Posture

Level of Difficulty: Intermediate

Step-by-Step Instructions:

- Sit on the mat with legs extended forward (Dandasana).
- Bend the right knee and bring the right foot onto the left thigh, sole facing upward.
- Bend the left knee and place the left foot onto the right thigh, sole facing upward.
- Adjust the knees so they are close to the floor and the spine remains tall and neutral.
- Rest the hands on the knees in Jnana Mudra (thumb and index finger touching).
- Relax the shoulders, close the eyes, and bring attention to the breath.
- Hold the posture for a few minutes, breathing naturally.
- To release, carefully unfold the legs one at a time.
- Repeat by switching the cross of the legs to balance both sides

Benefits:

- Enhances concentration and mental stability during meditation.
- Stretches the ankles, knees, and hips deeply.
- Promotes optimal alignment of the spine for prolonged sitting.
- Stimulates abdominal organs, aiding digestion.
- Calms the mind and helps awaken dormant energies.
-

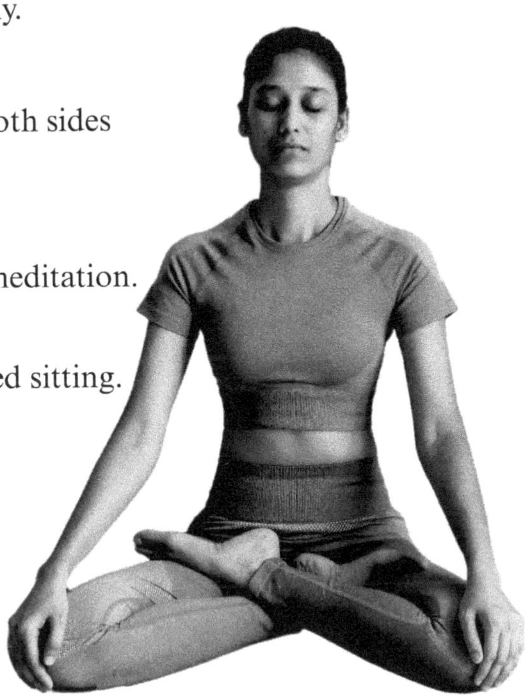

Padmasana

Contraindications:

- Avoid in case of knee, hip, or ankle injuries.
- Beginners should approach carefully to avoid forcing the legs.
- Not recommended for those with severe sciatica or lower back issues.

Modifications:

- Practice Ardha Padmasana (Half Lotus) if full Lotus is not accessible.
- Use a folded blanket or cushion under the hips to elevate and support the pelvis.

SIDDHASANA - Adepts Pose

Sanskrit Name: Siddhasana - सिद्धासन

English Name: Accomplished Pose

Category of Pose: Seated / Meditative

Level of Difficulty: Intermediate

Step-by-Step Instructions:

- Sit with both legs extended (Dandasana).
- Bend the left knee and bring the heel close to the perineum.
- Bend the right knee and place the right heel directly above the left heel, aligning it with the pubic bone.
- Allow toes to rest in the space between the calf and thigh muscles.
- Keep spine erect, chin slightly tucked, shoulders relaxed.
- Rest hands on knees in any comfortable mudra.
- Close the eyes and focus on breath or a point of meditation.

Benefits:

- Enhances concentration and mental stability during meditation.
- Stimulates the pelvic region and redirects energy upward.
- Strengthens the back and opens the hips gently.
- Promotes stillness and grounding in breathwork.

Contraindications:

- Severe knee or hip injuries.
- Discomfort in the ankles or tight groin.

Modifications:

- Use a cushion under the hips for elevation and comfort.
- Place a rolled towel or block under knees for support.
- Alternate legs over time to balance both sides.

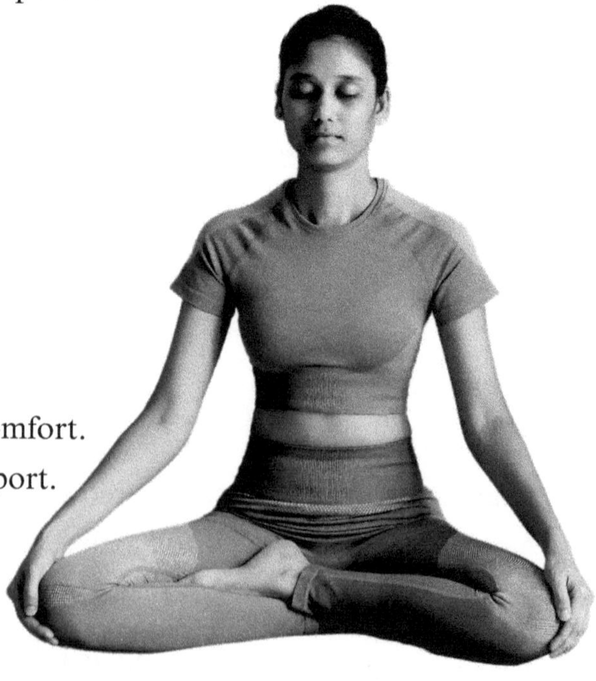

Siddhasana

VAJRASANA - Thunderbolt Pose

Sanskrit Name: Vajrasana - वज्रासन

English Name: Thunderbolt Pose / Diamond Pose

Category of Pose: Seated / Meditative / Digestive Support

Level of Difficulty: Beginner

Step-by-Step Instructions:

- Begin in a kneeling position with knees together and feet slightly apart.
- Sit back so that the buttocks rest on the heels, thighs resting on the calves.
- Keep spine straight, shoulders relaxed, and hands resting on thighs.
- Gaze forward or close the eyes, maintaining natural breath.

Benefits:

- Aids digestion and reduces bloating - ideal after meals.
- Calms the nervous system and supports meditative stillness.
- Strengthens lower back and pelvic muscles.
- Encourages better posture and alignment of the spine and hips.

Contraindications:

- Severe knee pain or recent surgery on the knees or ankles.
- Sciatica or spinal disc issues (modify with props).

Modifications:

- Place a folded blanket or cushion between hips and heels for comfort.
- Use a rolled towel under the ankles to reduce pressure.
- Practice for shorter durations, gradually increasing the time.

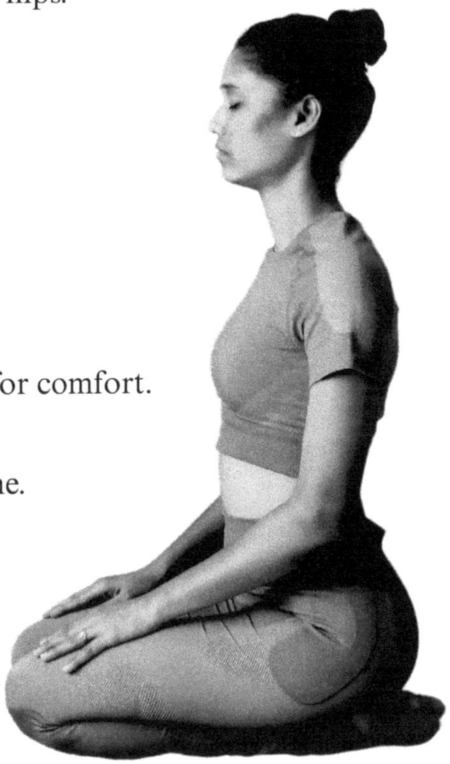

Vajrasana

USTRASANA - Camel Pose

Sanskrit Name: Ustrāsana - उष्ट्रासन

English Name: Camel Pose

Category of Pose: Kneeling Backbend

Level of Difficulty: Intermediate

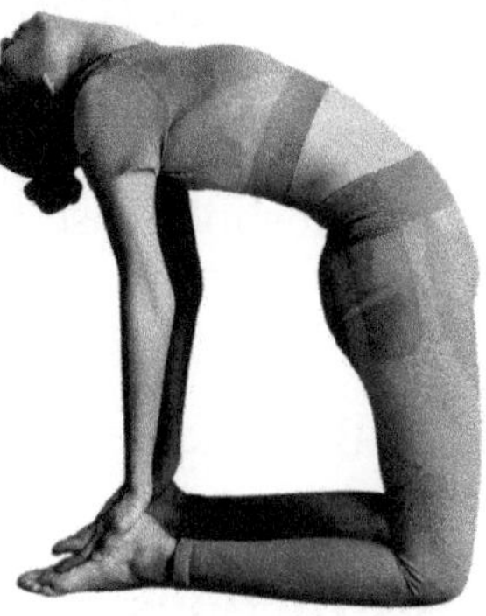

Ustrasana

Step-by-Step Instructions:

- Start with Vajrasana.
- Place your hands on your lower back with fingers pointing downward, supporting your spine.
- Inhale deeply, lift your chest, and begin to arch your back gently.
- Exhale, reach your hands back one at a time to hold your heels (toes tucked for beginners or flat for more intensity).
- Drop your head gently back if it feels comfortable, opening through the throat and chest.
- Hold the pose, breathing slowly for 20–30 seconds.
- To release, bring hands back to the hips, engage the core, and slowly return upright.

Benefits:

- Improves spinal flexibility and posture
- Strengthens the back, thighs, and glutes
- Opens the chest, lungs, abdomen, and hip flexors
- Stimulates digestive organs and improves elimination

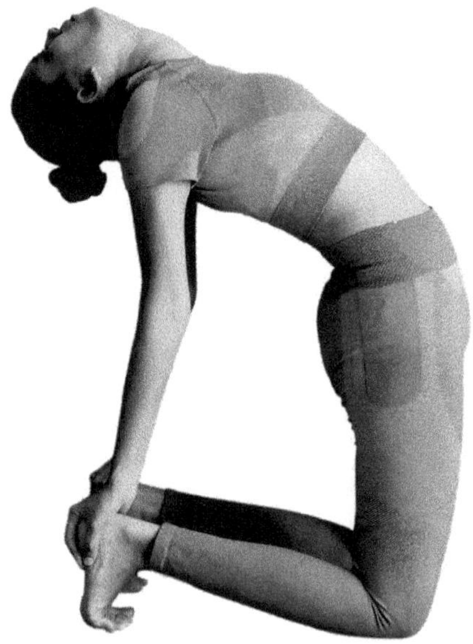

Ustrasana

Contraindications:

- Neck or back injuries, Hernia,
- High blood pressure, or severe headaches

Modifications:

- Place hands on lower back instead of heels for a gentler variation
- Tuck the toes to elevate the heels and reduce the backbend depth
- Use a yoga block on each side next to the heels for extra height/support

Counter Poses:

- Balasana (Child's Pose)

BALASANA - Child Pose

Sanskrit Name: Balasana - बालासन

English Name: Child's Pose

Category of Pose: Restorative / Prone / Forward Bend

Level of Difficulty: Beginner

Step-by-Step Instructions:

- Start in a kneeling position, big toes touching, knees together or hip-width apart.
- Sit back on the heels and slowly fold the torso forward.
- Extend arms forward (**Active Child Pose**) or alongside the body (**Resting Child Pose**).
- Allow the forehead to rest on the mat, relaxing the neck and shoulders.
- Breathe deeply, allowing the back to expand with each inhale.

Benefits:

- Gently stretches hips, thighs, and lower back.
- Calms the mind and reduces stress or fatigue.
- Supports digestion and soothes abdominal organs.
- Offers rest and integration between active poses.

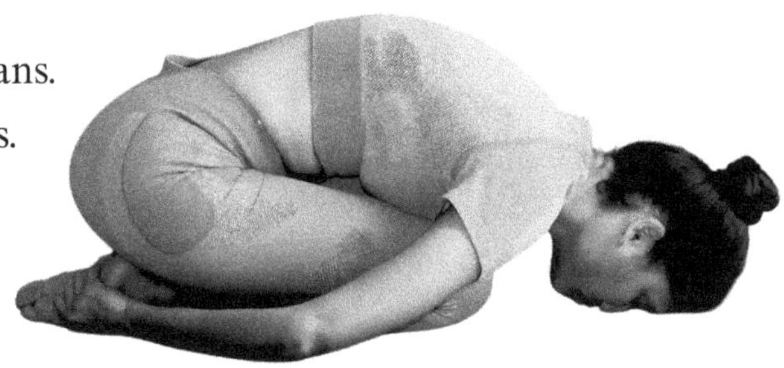

Balasana

Contraindications:

- Knee injuries or severe ankle pain.
- Recent abdominal surgery (avoid deep forward folding).

Modifications:

- Place a cushion under the torso or forehead.
- Use a folded blanket under the hips or ankles for added support.
- Spread knees wider for deeper release or comfort.

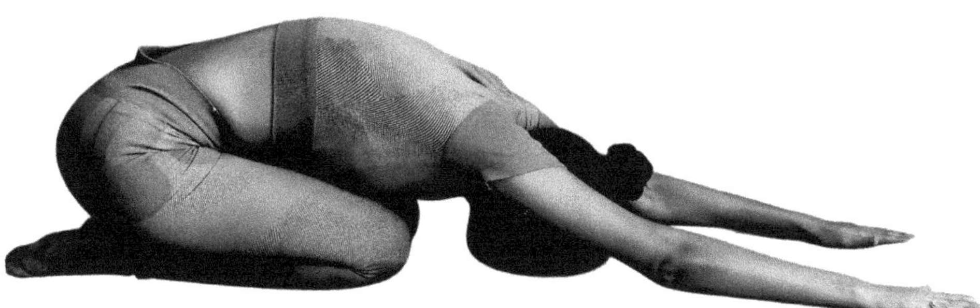

Balasana

BADDHA KONASANA - Bound Angle Pose

Sanskrit Name: Baddha Konasana - बद्ध कोणासन

English Name: Bound Angle Pose / Cobbler's Pose

Category of Pose: Seated / Hip-Opener

Level of Difficulty: Beginner

Step-by-Step Instructions:

- Sit in Dandasana with legs extended.
- Bend both knees and bring the soles of the feet together.
- Let the knees fall out to the sides like butterfly wings.
- Hold the feet or ankles with both hands.
- Keep the spine upright and shoulders relaxed.
- For a deeper stretch, gently press the knees toward the floor without force.

Benefits:

- Open the hips and groin gently and effectively.
- Stimulates abdominal organs, bladder, and kidneys.
- Supports reproductive and digestive systems.
- Calms the nervous system and helps reduce fatigue.

Contraindications:

- Severe hip or knee injuries.
- Recent groin or lower back surgery

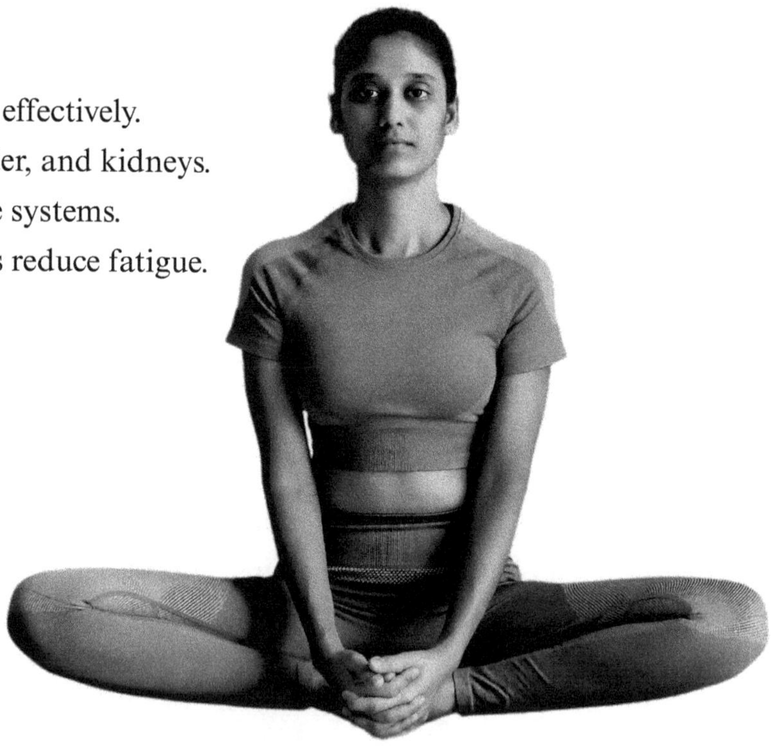

Baddha Konasana

Modifications:

- Place cushions or blocks under each knee for support.
- Sit on a folded blanket to elevate the hips.

PASCHIMOTTANASANA – Seated Forward Bend

Sanskrit Name: Paschimottanasana - पश्चिमोत्तानासन

English Name: Seated Forward Bend

Category of Pose: Seated / Forward Bend

Level of Difficulty: Beginner to Intermediate

Step-by-Step Instructions:

- Begin seated in Dandasana (Staff Pose), legs extended and together.
- Inhale and raise the arms overhead, lengthening the spine.
- Exhale and hinge forward from the hips, keeping the spine long.
- Reach hands toward the feet, grasp the toes, sides of the feet, or shins.
- Let the head and neck relax gently, staying mindful not to round the lower back excessively.
- Breathe deeply and stay in the pose for 5–8 breaths, gradually increasing duration over time.

Benefits:

- Stretches the entire back body, spine, hamstrings, and calves.
- Stimulates abdominal organs and aids digestion.
- Calms the nervous system, reduces anxiety, and relieves stress.
- Improves flexibility and strengthens mental focus.

Contraindications:

- Herniated discs or acute lower back pain.
- Asthma or respiratory difficulties (avoid compressing the chest deeply).
- Hamstring or hip injuries.

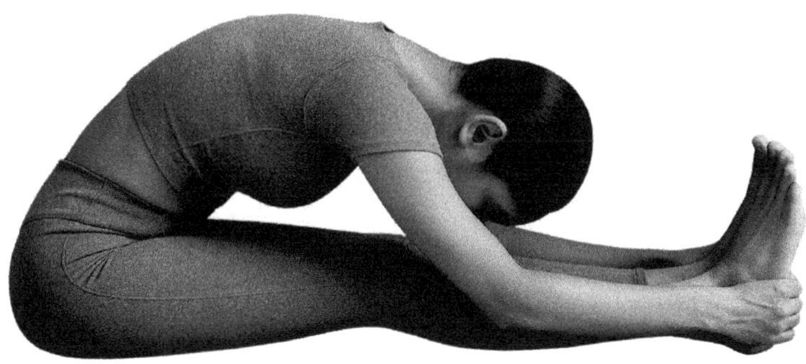

Paschimottanasana

Modifications:

- Sit on a folded blanket to elevate the hips for better pelvic tilt.
- Use a yoga strap around the feet if flexibility is limited.
- Bend the knees slightly to protect the lower back and hamstrings.

JANU SIRSASANA – Head-to-Knee Pose

Sanskrit Name: Janu Sirsasana - जानु शीर्षासन

English Name: Head-to-Knee Forward Bend

Category of Pose: Seated / Forward Bend

Level of Difficulty: Beginner to Intermediate

Step-by-Step Instructions:

- Begin seated in Dandasana (Staff Pose).
- Bend the right knee and bring the sole of the right foot to the inner left thigh.
- Inhale, raise both arms overhead, lengthening the spine.
- Exhale, hinge forward from the hips over the extended left leg, bringing the forehead toward the left knee
- Reach hands to the foot, shin, or use a strap if needed.
- Allow the spine to stay long and the head to relax.
- Stay for 5–10 breaths, then inhale to come up and repeat on the other side.

Benefits:

- Deeply stretches the hamstrings, spine, and lower back.
- Stimulates the liver, kidneys, and digestive system.
- Calms the mind and reduces anxiety.
- Supports detoxification and menstrual health.

Contraindications:

- Severe lower back injury.
- Recent hamstring tears.

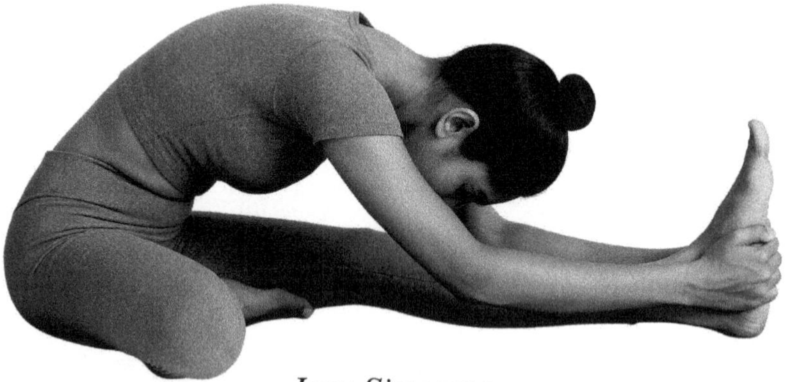

Janu Sirsasana

Modifications:

- Sit on a folded blanket to ease hip tightness.
- Use a strap around the extended foot if you cannot reach comfortably.
- Place a cushion under the bent knee for support if it doesn't touch the ground.

ARDHA MATSYENDRASANA – Half Lord of the Fishes

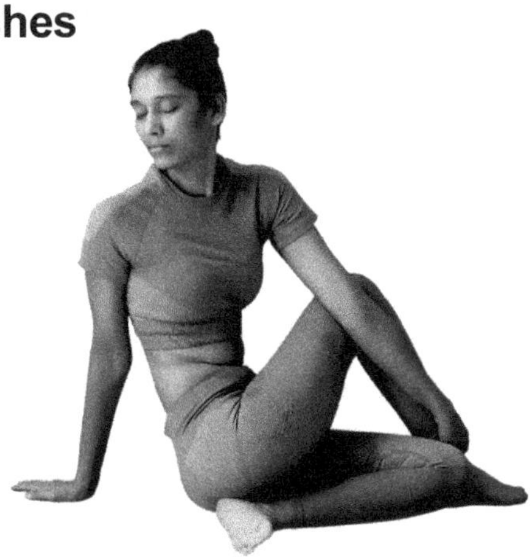

Ardha Matsyendrasana

Sanskrit Name: Ardha Matsyendrasana - अर्ध मत्स्येन्द्रासन

English Name: Half Lord of the Fishes Pose

Category of Pose: Seated / Twist

Level of Difficulty: Intermediate

Step-by-Step Instructions:

- Sit in Dandasana (Staff Pose).
- Bend the right knee and place the right foot flat on the floor outside the left thigh.
- Bend the left leg and tuck the left foot near the right hip.
- Inhale, lengthen the spine.
- Exhale, twist to the right, placing the right hand behind you and the left elbow outside the right knee.
- Keep the chest open, spine tall, and shoulders relaxed.
- Look over the right shoulder if comfortable.
- Hold for 5–8 breaths, then gently release and repeat on the other side.

Benefits:

- Deeply massages abdominal organs, stimulates digestion, and promotes detoxification.
- Enhances spinal flexibility and tones spinal nerves.
- Opens the chest and shoulders, aiding respiratory function.
- Relieves lower back tension and improves posture.

Contraindications:

- Herniated discs or recent spinal injuries.
- Post-abdominal surgery (avoid strong compression).

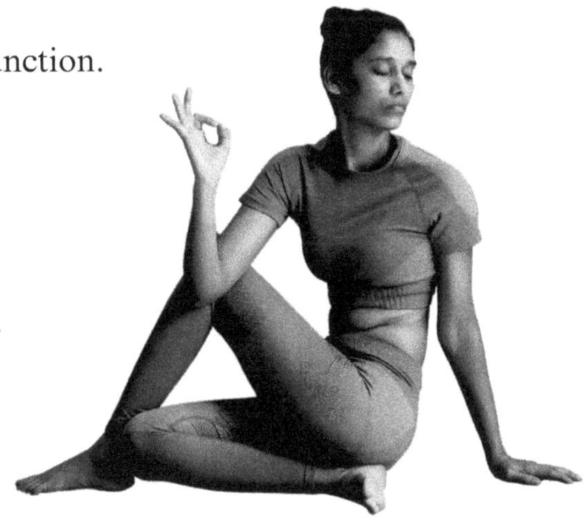

Ardha Matsyendrasana

Modifications:

- Keep the bottom leg extended if the hips or knees feel strained.
- Use a block under the supporting hand to maintain lift in the spine.

GOMUKHASANA – Cow Face Pose

Sanskrit Name: Gomukhasana - गोमुखासन

English Name: Cow Face Pose

Category of Pose: Seated / Hip Opener

Level of Difficulty: Intermediate

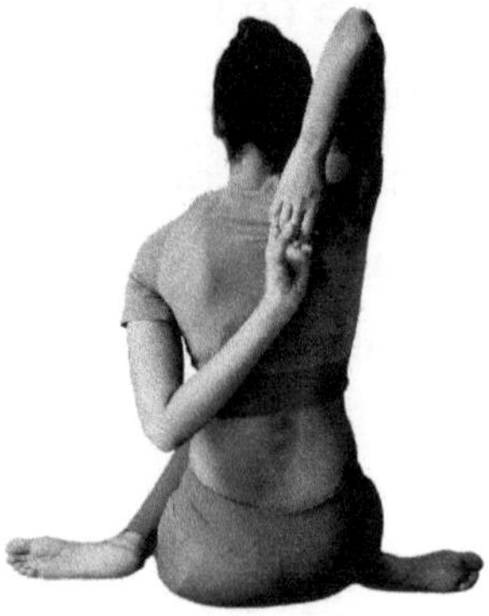

Gomukhasana

Step-by-Step Instructions:

- Sit in Dandasana (Staff Pose).
- Bend the left knee and bring the left foot under the right thigh beside the right hip.
- Cross the right leg over the left, stacking the right knee directly above the left.
- Bring the right arm up and bend the elbow, reaching down the back.
- Bring the left arm behind the back and try to clasp hands.
- Keep the spine tall and chest open.
- **Advanced -** bend forward, bringing forehead toward the knee
- Hold for 5–8 breaths, then switch sides.

Benefits:

- Deeply stretches hips, thighs, ankles, shoulders, and chest.
- Improves posture and upper body mobility.
- Releases tension in the hips and shoulders from long sitting or stress.
- Stimulates kidney and reproductive organ function.

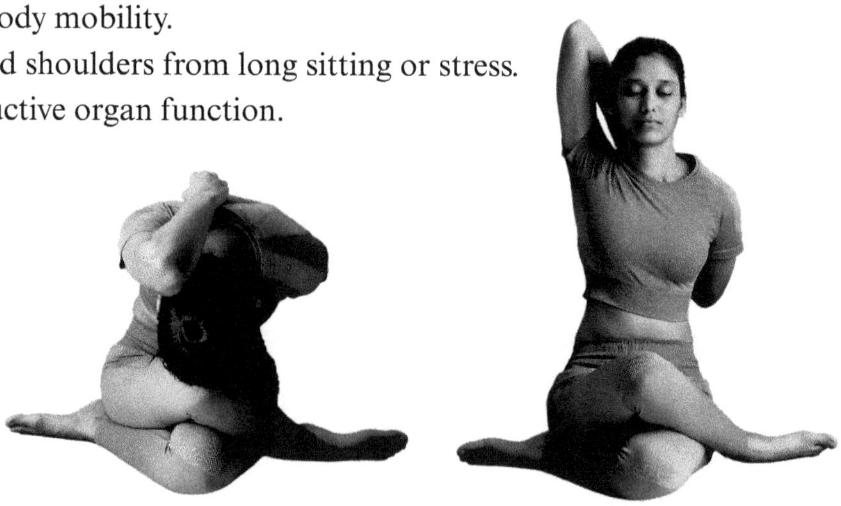

Gomukhasana

Contraindications:

- Severe shoulder, knee, or hip injuries.
- Frozen shoulder (modify arm movement).

Modifications:

- Use a strap between the hands if they don't clasp comfortably.
- If legs don't stack evenly, keep the bottom leg extended.

NAVASANA – Boat Pose

Sanskrit Name: Navasana - नावासन

English Name: Boat Pose

Category of Pose: Seated / Core Strengthening

Level of Difficulty: Intermediate

Step-by-Step Instructions:

- Sit in Dandasana (Staff Pose) with legs extended and spine straight.
- Bend the knees slightly, place hands behind the thighs for support.
- Lean back slightly, keeping the spine long, not rounded.
- Lift the feet off the floor, shins parallel to the mat.
- Extend arms forward parallel to the floor, palms facing in.
- For full expression, straighten the legs to a **"V"** shape.
- Keep the chest lifted and engage the core. Hold for 3–5 breaths.
- Slowly lower the legs and rest.

Benefits:

- Strengthens the core, hip flexors, and spine.
- Improves balance and coordination.
- Stimulates digestion and abdominal organs.
- Builds focus and stamina.

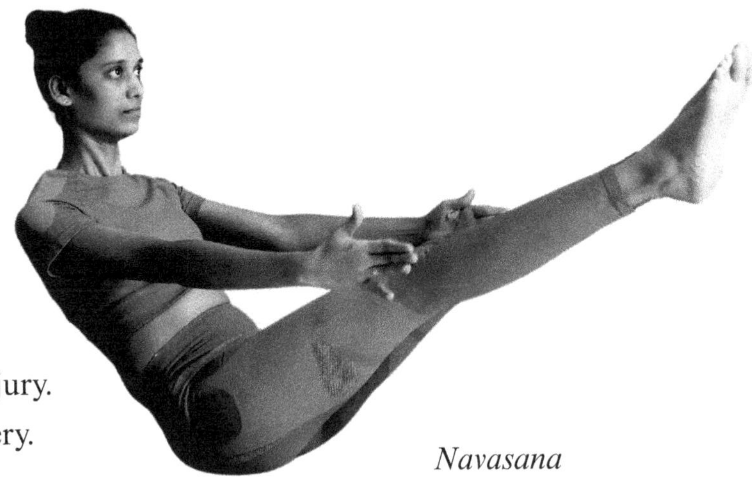

Navasana

Contraindications:

- Lower back pain or recent spinal injury.
- Hernia or abdominal surgery recovery.

Modifications:

- Keep knees bent or feet on the floor to reduce strain.
- Hold behind the thighs if core strength is limited.
- Place a strap under the soles of the feet to support extended legs.

CHAKKI CHALANASANA – Churning the Mill

Sanskrit Name: Chakki Chalanasana - चक्की चलनासन

English Name: Churning the Mill Pose

Category of Pose: Seated / Dynamic Yogic Movement (Sukshma Vyayama)

Level of Difficulty: Beginner

Step-by-Step Instructions:

- Sit with legs stretched wide apart, feet flexed.
- Interlock fingers and extend the arms straight forward at chest level.
- Inhale deeply.
- Begin rotating the arms forward in a large circular motion over the legs, as if churning a millstone.
- Exhale as you go forward, inhale as you come back.
- Perform 8–10 rounds clockwise, then repeat counterclockwise.
- Keep the spine active, avoid collapsing the chest.

Benefits:

- Loosens and strengthens the lower back, hips, abdomen, and thighs.
- Enhances digestive functions and massages abdominal organs.
- Increases hip joint mobility.
- Gently warms up the spine and prepares the body for deeper asanas.

Contraindications:

- Severe lower back pain or slipped disc.
- Recent abdominal surgery.

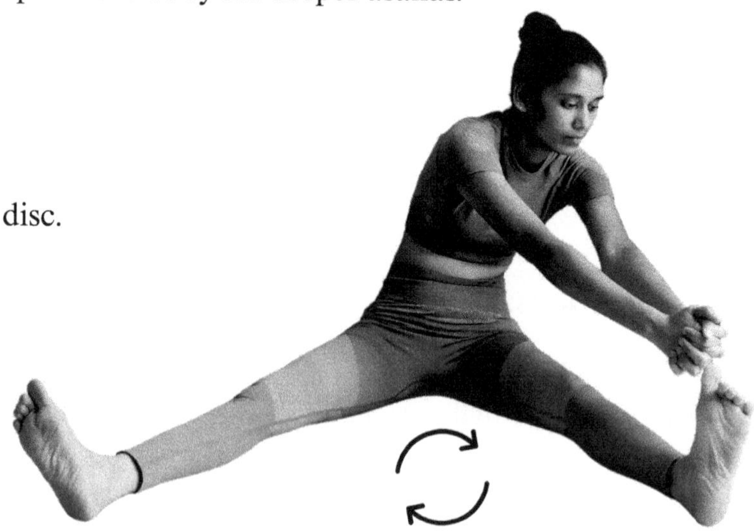

Chakki Chalanasana

Modifications:

- Keep the circle smaller to reduce intensity or range.

Standing Yoga Asanas

SAMASTHITI – Equal Standing Pose

Sanskrit Name: Samasthiti - समस्थितिः

English Name: Equal Standing Pose / Mountain Pose (in some schools)

Category of Pose: Standing / Foundational

Level of Difficulty: Beginner

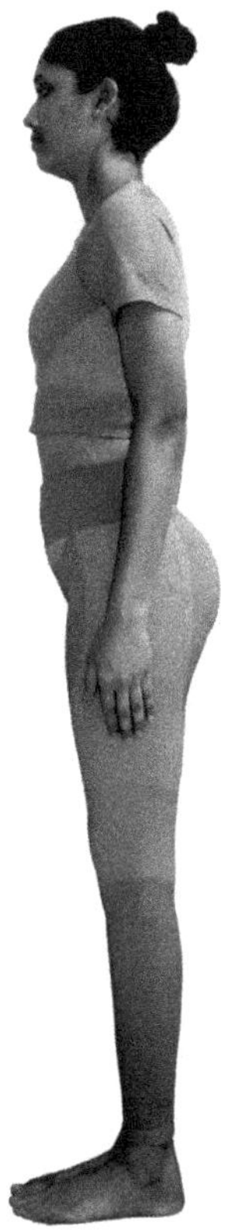

Samasthiti

Step-by-Step Instructions:

- Stand with feet together or hip-width apart, toes pointing forward.
- Distribute weight evenly on both feet - heels and toes grounded.
- Engage the thighs without locking the knees.
- Tuck the tailbone slightly and lengthen through the spine.
- Roll shoulders back and down; arms relaxed alongside the body.
- Palms can face the body or forward.
- Keep the neck long and chin parallel to the floor.
- Gaze softly straight ahead. Breathe naturally and stand with awareness.

Benefits:

- Cultivates posture awareness and balance.
- Enhances body alignment and grounding.
- Improves concentration and calm presence.
- Prepares mind and body for yoga practice.

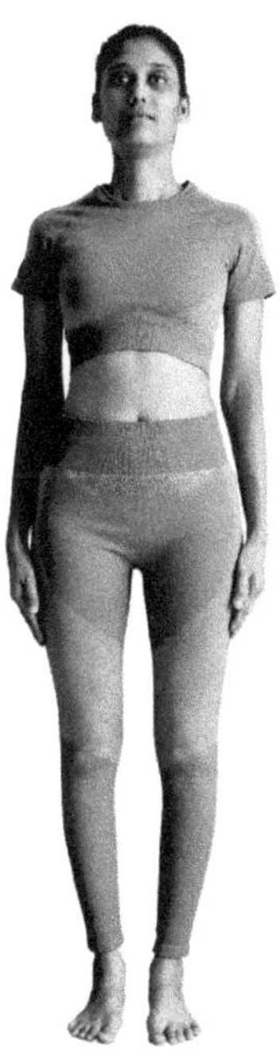

Samasthiti

TADASANA – Mountain Pose

Sanskrit Name: Tadasana - ताडासन

English Name: Mountain Pose

Category of Pose: Standing / Foundational

Level of Difficulty: Beginner

Step-by-Step Instructions:

- Start with Samasthiti, stand upright with feet together or hip-width apart, toes pointing forward.
- Interlock fingers in front; inhale and raise the arms overhead, turning palms upward.
- Lift heels off the floor, balancing on the balls of the feet.
- Keep arms straight alongside the ears, shoulders relaxed and drawn down.
- Neck stays long, chin parallel, gaze forward or slightly upward.
- Breathe deeply and hold for 5–8 breaths, maintaining stability.
- Exhale to lower the heels and arms gently, returning to neutral standing.

Benefits:

- Enhances postural alignment and body awareness
- Improves balance and coordination
- Strengthens the legs, calves, ankles, and core stability
- Promotes mindful breathing and grounding
- Prepares the body and mind for other standing poses

Contraindications:

- Severe balance disorders (use wall support).
- Low blood pressure (rise slowly if feeling lightheaded).

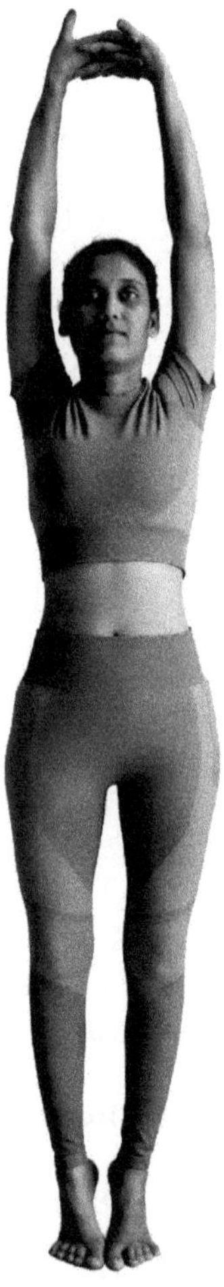

Tadasana

Modifications:

- Avoid heel lifting in case of severe balance disorders
- If interlocking the fingers is uncomfortable, simply raise the arms separately with palms facing each other

PADAHASTASANA – Hand-to-Foot Pose

Sanskrit Name: Padahastasana - पादहस्तासन

English Name: Hand Under Foot Pose

Category of Pose: Standing / Forward Bend

Level of Difficulty: Beginner to Intermediate

Step-by-Step Instructions:

- Start in Samasthiti, feet hip-width apart.
- Inhale and raise the arms overhead to lengthen the spine.
- Exhale and hinge from the hips to fold forward, bringing your chest toward your thighs.
- Slide both hands under the feet, palms facing up, toes meeting the wrists.
- Keep a gentle bend in the knees if hamstrings are tight.
- Relax the head and neck, letting the crown drop down.
- Engage the thighs slightly and press the feet into the hands.
- Breathe deeply, holding for 5–8 breaths, then release hands and slowly rise on an inhale.

Benefits:

- Stretches the hamstrings, calves, and lower back.
- Improves digestion and massages internal organs.
- Calms the mind and reduces stress.
- Enhances the flexibility of the spine and legs.
- Stimulates the nervous system.

Contraindications:

- Severe lower back pain or disc issues.
- High blood pressure or glaucoma.

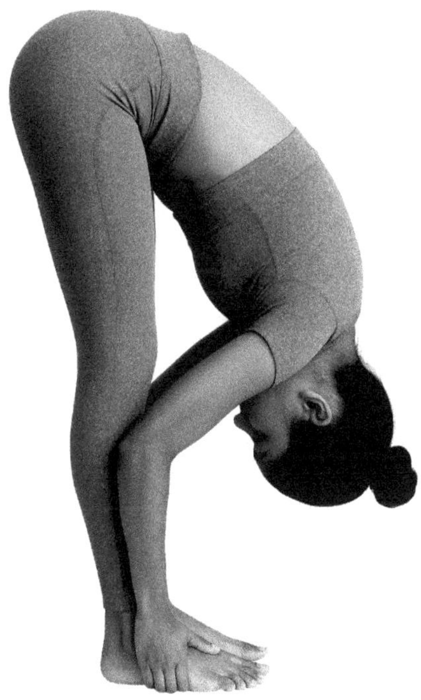

Padahastasana

Modifications:

- Perform with blocks under hands for a gentler version
- Use a strap around the feet if hands can't reach under them.
- Slightly bend the knees to avoid strain on the hamstrings or lower back.

TRIKONASANA – Triangle Pose

Sanskrit Name: Trikoṇāsana - त्रिकोणासन

English Name: Triangle Pose

Category of Pose: Standing / Lateral Bend

Level of Difficulty: Beginner

Step-by-Step Instructions:

- Begin standing in Samasthiti, then step the feet about 3–4 feet apart.
- Turn the right foot out 90° and the left foot slightly in, aligning the right heel with the left arch.
- Extend arms out to the sides at shoulder height, palms facing down.
- Inhale to lengthen the spine.
- Exhale, reach the right hand forward, and tilt the torso over the right leg.
- Place the right hand on the shin, ankle, or a block; extend the left arm straight up.
- Keep both legs active, chest open, and spine long.
- Gaze up at the top hand (or down if neck sensitivity).
- Hold for 5–8 breaths, then inhale to rise back up and switch sides.

Benefits:

- Stretches and strengthens the legs, hips, and spine.
- Opens the chest and shoulders.
- Improves digestion and stimulates abdominal organs.
- Enhances balance and body awareness.
- Alleviates backache and stress.

Contraindications:

- Neck or back injury
- Hyperextension in the knee.

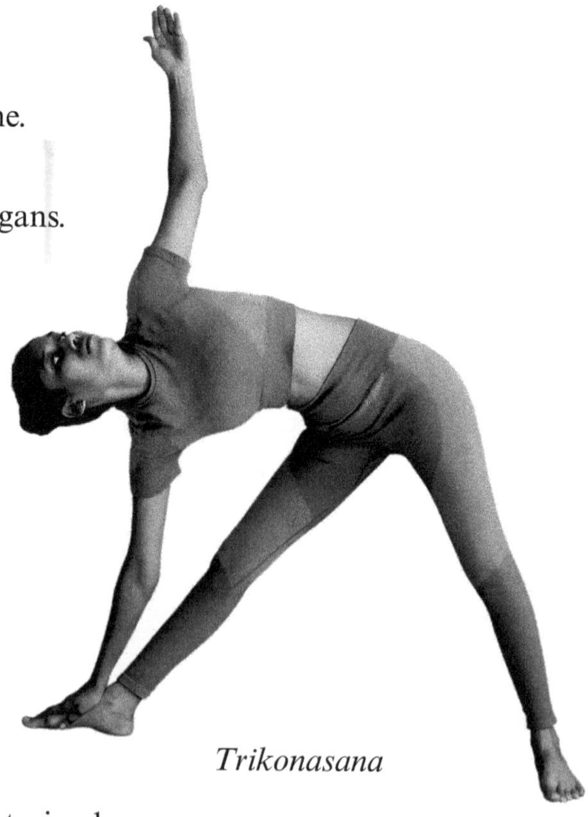

Trikonasana

Modifications:

- Gaze downward or straight ahead if the neck is strained.
- Use a block under the bottom hand to maintain proper alignment.

VRIKSHASANA – Tree Pose

Sanskrit Name: Vrikshasana - वृक्षासन

English Name: Tree Pose

Category of Pose: Standing / Balancing

Level of Difficulty: Beginner to Intermediate

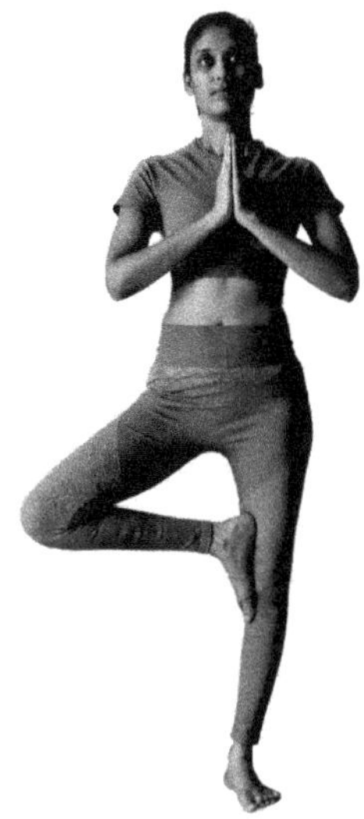

Vrikshasana

Step-by-Step Instructions:

- Begin in Samasthiti.
- Shift weight onto the left foot, grounding it firmly.
- Bend the right knee and place the sole of the right foot:
  - **Beginners**: on the ankle or calf (avoid the knee).
  - **Advanced**: on the inner left thigh, pressing firmly.
- Bring palms together at the heart center (Anjali Mudra) or raise arms overhead, shoulders relaxed.
- Gaze softly at a fixed point in front for balance.
- Hold the position for 5–10 breaths, then slowly release and switch sides.

Benefits:

- Improves balance, concentration, and body awareness.
- Strengthens legs, ankles, and core muscles.
- Stretches inner thighs, groins, and shoulders.
- Cultivates focus and a calm mind.

Contraindications:

- Vertigo or severe balance issues.
- Knee or ankle injuries.

Modifications:

- Use a wall or chair for balance support.
- Keep toes on the floor with the heel at the ankle for stability.
- Hold the pose for shorter durations if new to balancing postures.

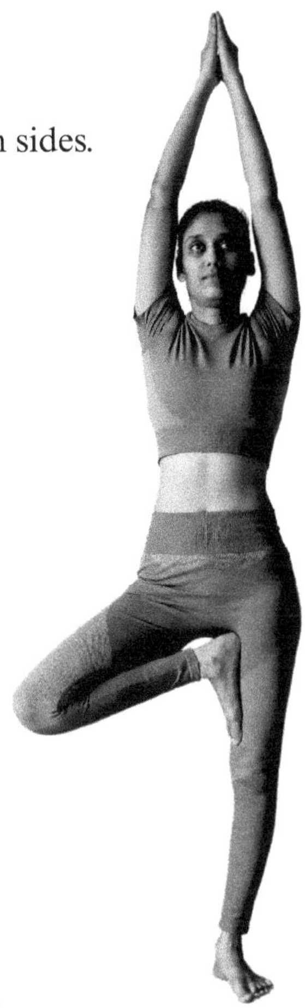

Vrikshasana

NATARAJASANA – Dancer's Pose

Sanskrit Name: Natarajasana - नटराजासन

English Name: Dancer's Pose

Category of Pose: Standing / Balancing / Backbend

Level of Difficulty: Intermediate

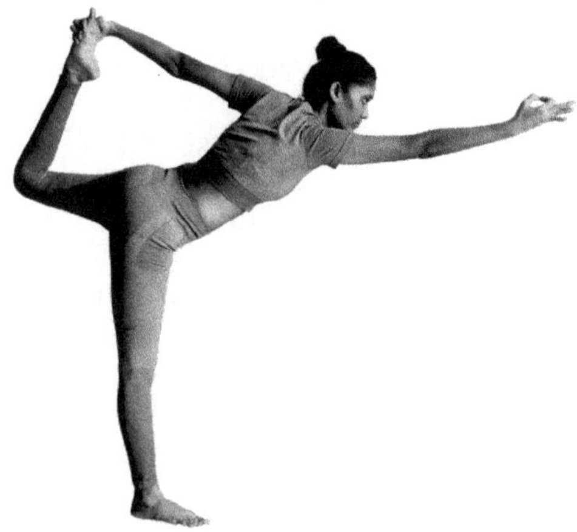

Natrajasana

Step-by-Step Instructions:

- Start in Samasthiti, standing tall and centered.
- Shift weight onto the left foot.
- Bend the right knee and bring the right heel toward the buttocks.
- Reach the right hand back to grasp the inside of the right foot or ankle.
- Inhale and extend the left arm forward at shoulder height, palm facing down.
- On an exhale, press the right foot into the hand to lift the leg behind while slightly hinging forward from the hips.
- Keep the chest lifted and hips squared as much as possible.
- Focus the gaze on a steady point to maintain balance.
- Hold for 3–5 breaths, then slowly release and switch sides.

Benefits:

- Enhances balance, focus, and grace.
- Strengthens legs, ankles, back, and shoulders.
- Stretches the chest, hip flexors, and thighs.
- Opens the heart and improves posture.

Contraindications:

- Knee issues (avoid pulling the foot forcefully).
- Shoulder instability, Low back injuries, or chronic pain.

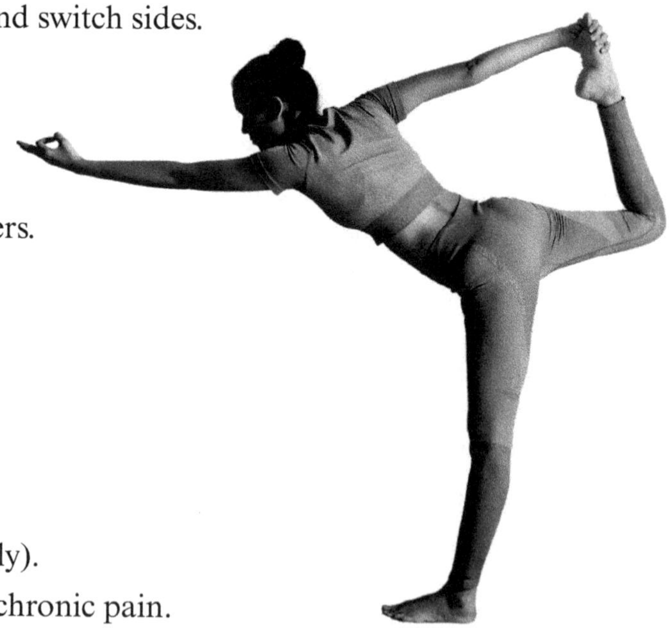

Natrajasana

Modifications:

- Use a wall or chair for balance support.
- Hold a strap looped around the lifted foot if reaching the ankle is difficult.

MALASANA – Garland Pose

Sanskrit Name: Malāsana - मालासन

English Name: Garland Pose

Category of Pose: Standing / Hip Opener / Grounding

Level of Difficulty: Beginner

Step-by-Step Instructions:

- Start in Samasthiti with feet slightly wider than hips.
- Turn feet out slightly and begin to bend the knees, coming into a deep squat.
- Bring the hips down toward the heels; keep heels grounded (or use support if they lift).
- Bring palms together at the heart in Anjali Mudra (Namaskar), using elbows to gently press the knees open.
- Lift the chest, lengthen the spine, and draw the shoulders away from the ears.
- Gaze forward or softly downward.
- Hold for 5–10 breaths, breathing deeply into the hips and lower back.

Benefits:

- Opens the hips, groin, and ankles.
- Improves digestion and elimination.
- Strengthens the lower back and pelvic floor.
- Grounds energy and improves balance.

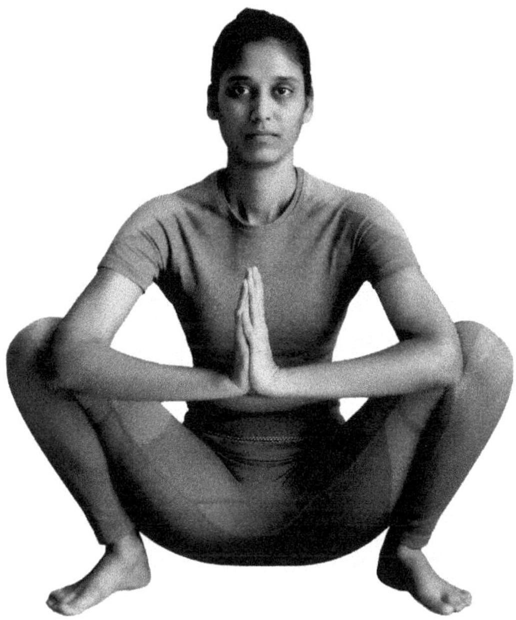

Malasana

Contraindications:

- Knee or ankle injuries - approach with caution or modify.
- Severe lower back issues - use support or avoid deep squatting.

Modifications:

- Place a rolled blanket or block under the heels if they don't touch the ground.
- Sit on a block if squatting deeply is uncomfortable.
- Keep hands on the floor for extra support and balance.

Supine Yoga Asanas - Lying on the Back

SAVASANA – Corpse Pose

Sanskrit Name: Śavāsana - शवासन

English Name: Corpse Pose

Category of Pose: Supine / Restorative / Meditative

Level of Difficulty: Beginner

Step-by-Step Instructions:

- Lie flat on your back, arms resting at the sides with palms facing up.
- Extend your legs straight, allowing feet to fall naturally outward.
- Close the eyes gently and relax the entire body.
- Breathe slowly, evenly, and naturally.
- Release all muscular tension from head to toe.
- Let the body surrender to the floor, mentally scanning to relax each part.
- Stay in the pose for 1–2 minutes, or longer as needed.

Benefits:

- Deeply relaxes the body and calms the nervous system.
- Reduces stress, anxiety, and fatigue.
- Promotes integration of the practice and mental clarity.
- Lowers blood pressure and supports overall healing.

Contraindications: Back discomfort

Modifications:

- Place a bolster or rolled blanket under the knees for lower back support.

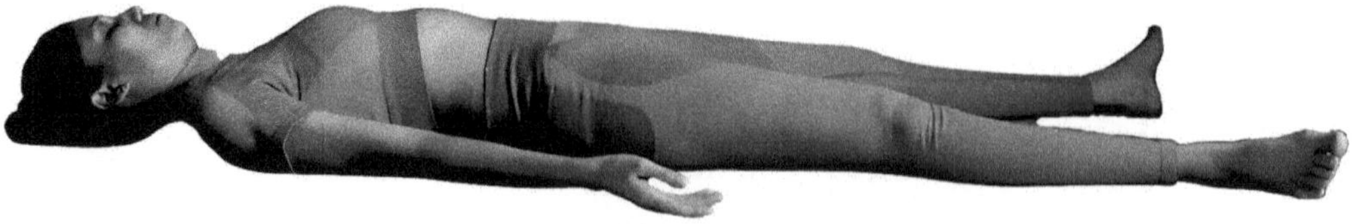

Savasana

UTTANPADASANA – Raised Leg Pose

Sanskrit Name: Uttānapādāsana - उत्तानपादासन

English Name: Raised Leg Pose

Category of Pose: Supine / Core Strengthening

Level of Difficulty: Beginner to Intermediate

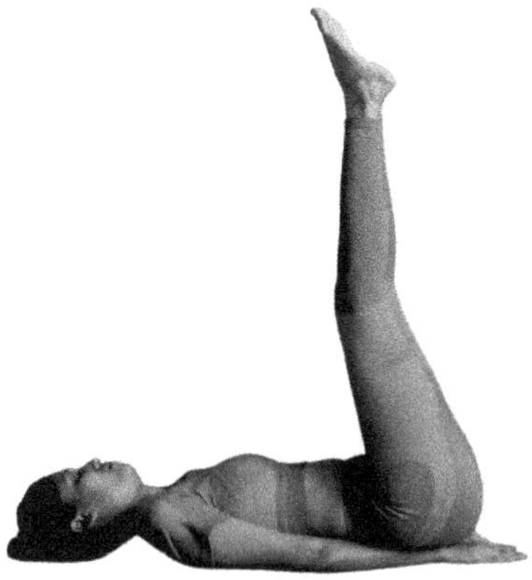

Uttanapadasana

Step-by-Step Instructions:

- Lie comfortably on your back, legs extended, arms beside your body, palms facing down.
- Inhale deeply. As you exhale, engage the abdominal muscles and slowly lift both legs up to about 60 to 90 degrees, keeping them straight.
- Keep the lower back grounded, neck relaxed, and avoid straining.
- Hold the posture for 5–10 breaths, maintaining steady, even breathing.
- To release, exhale, and slowly lower the legs back to the ground without jerking.
- Rest in Savasana or with bent knees briefly before repeating.

Benefits:

- Strengthens the core muscles, hip flexors, and lower back.
- Stimulates the abdominal organs and improves digestion.
- Tones the legs and enhances control over lower body movement.
- Improves energy and blood flow, especially in the pelvic region.

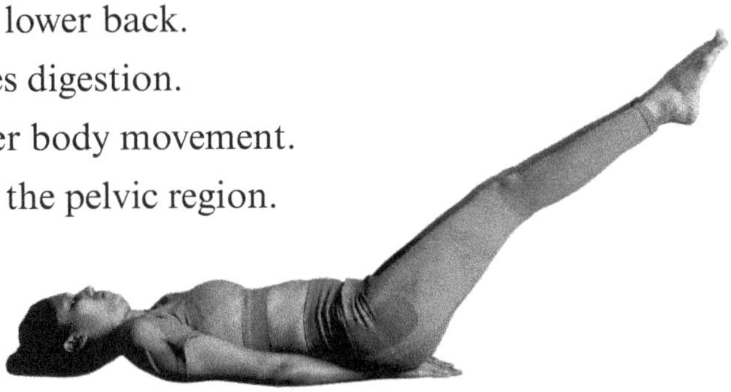

Contraindications:

- Lower back pain or spinal issues
- High blood pressure or hernia

Modifications:

- Beginners can raise one leg at a time for ease and safety.
- Keep the legs slightly bent if the hamstrings are tight.
- Place hands under the hips for lumbar support.

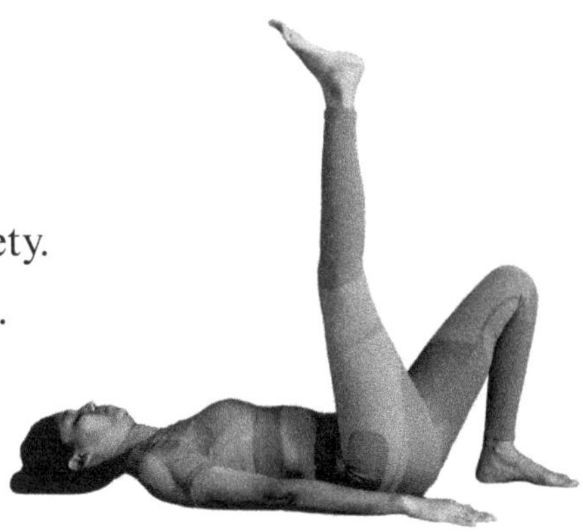

Ekapada Uttanapadasana

PAVANAMUKTASANA – Wind-Relieving Pose

Sanskrit Name: Pavanamuktāsana - पवनमुक्तासन

English Name: Wind-Relieving Pose

Category of Pose: Supine / Digestive / Relaxation

Level of Difficulty: Beginner

Step-by-Step Instructions:

- Lie comfortably on your back, legs extended, arms by your sides.
- Inhale. As you exhale, bend both knees and draw them towards your chest.
- Wrap your arms around your shins, clasping opposite elbows or wrists.
- Gently press the thighs into the abdomen, keeping your back flat on the floor.
- Optionally, lift the head and chin toward the knees, maintaining a soft gaze.
- Breathe slowly and hold the posture for 5–10 breaths.
- To release, lower your head (if lifted), then slowly extend the legs back to the mat.

Benefits:

- Relieves gas, bloating, and constipation.
- Gently stretches the lower back and hips.
- Helps release tension and calm the nervous system.
- Stimulates the digestive system and supports abdominal organ health.

Contraindications:

- Recent abdominal surgery, hernia, or spinal injuries.

Modifications:

- Keep the head down if there's neck strain.
- Hug one knee at a time (Ekapada Pawanmuktasana) for more ease or for beginners.

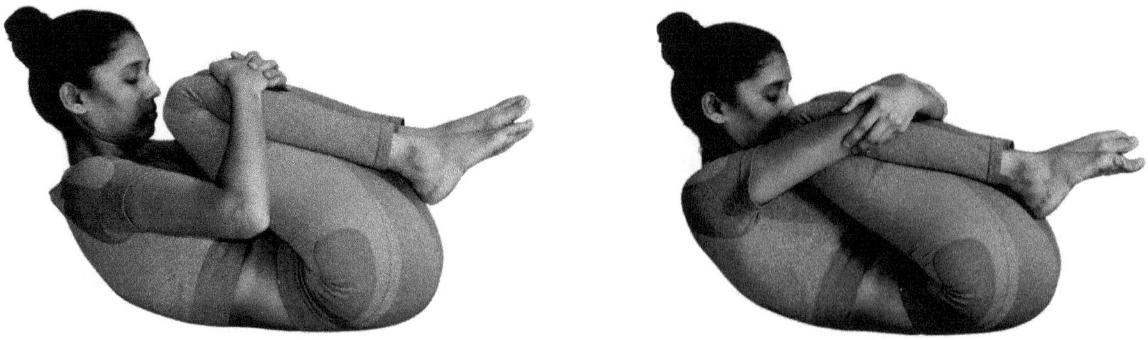

Pavanamuktasana

EKAPADA PAVANAMUKTASANA – One-Legged Wind-Relieving Pose

Sanskrit Name: Ekapāda Pawanmuktasana - एकपाद पवनमुक्तासन

English Name: One-Legged Wind-Relieving Pose

Category of Pose: Supine / Relaxation / Digestive

Level of Difficulty: Beginner

Step-by-Step Instructions:

- Lie on your back with legs extended and arms resting by your sides.
- Inhale deeply. As you exhale, bend the right knee and draw it toward your chest.
- Interlace your fingers over the shin or behind the thigh.
- Keep the left leg extended and relaxed on the floor.
- Gently press the thigh into the abdomen without straining the neck or shoulders.
- Keep the shoulders grounded, spine neutral, and breathe steadily.
- Hold for 5–10 breaths, then exhale and release the leg.
- Repeat on the left side.

Benefits:

- Stimulates the digestive system and relieves gas and bloating.
- Gently massages the abdominal organs.
- Releases tension in the lower back and hips.
- Calms the mind and supports relaxation.

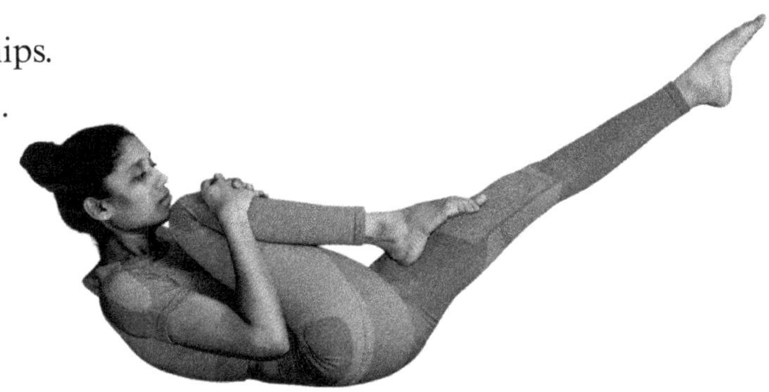

Contraindications:

- Recent abdominal surgery or hernia.

Modifications:

- Use a strap behind the thigh if reaching the shin is difficult.
- Place a small cushion under the head or lower back for support.

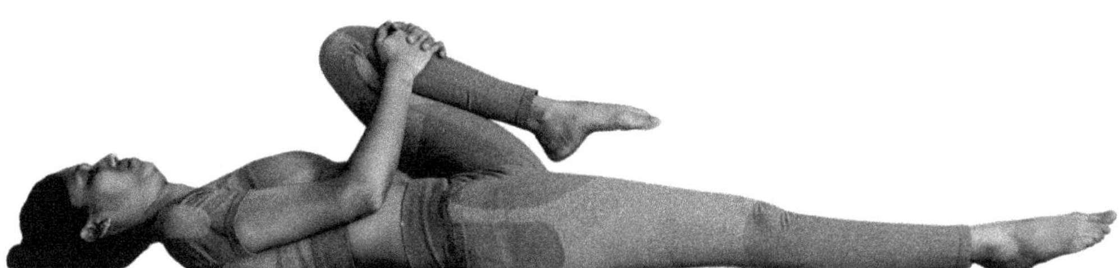

Ekapada Pavanamuktasana

SETU BANDHASANA – Bridge Pose

Sanskrit Name: Setu Bandhāsana - सेतु बन्धासन

English Name: Bridge Pose

Category of Pose: Supine / Backbend

Level of Difficulty: Beginner to Intermediate

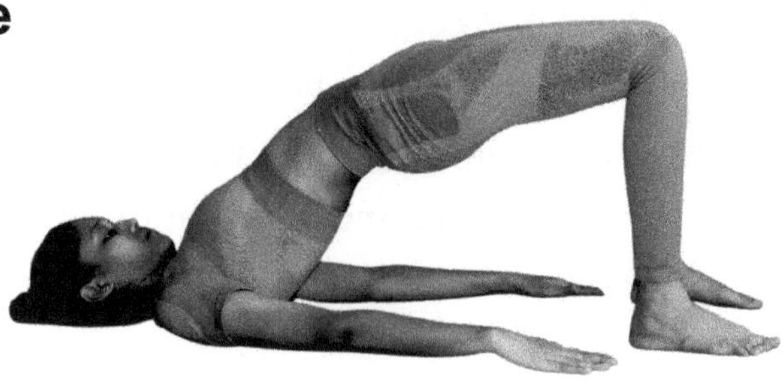

Setu Bandhasana

Step-by-Step Instructions:

- Lie on your back with knees bent and feet hip-width apart, flat on the floor close to the sitting bones.
- Keep your arms alongside the body, palms facing down.
- Inhale deeply. As you exhale, press into the feet and lift your hips upward.
- Tuck the shoulders slightly underneath and interlace the hands beneath your back (optional).
- Engage the glutes, thighs, and core, keeping knees in line with the ankles.
- Avoid turning the head; keep the neck long and gaze up.
- Hold for 5–10 breaths, then exhale and gently roll down to the mat.

Benefits:

- Strengthens the glutes, hamstrings, and lower back.
- Stretches the chest, neck, and spine.
- Stimulates the thyroid gland and abdominal organs.
- Reduces anxiety and fatigue, and may relieve menstrual discomfort.

Contraindications:

- Recent or chronic **neck, spine, or shoulder injuries**.
- Uncontrolled **high blood pressure** or severe migraines

Modifications:

- Place a block under the sacrum for a restorative variation.
- Keep the arms extended flat if shoulder mobility is limited.
- Use a **strap around the thighs** to prevent the knees from splaying.

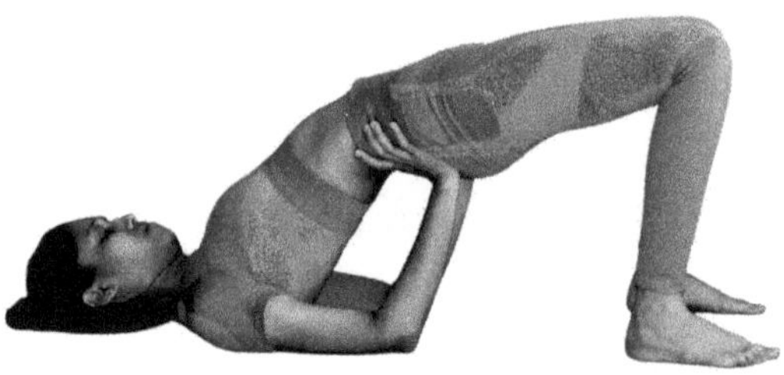

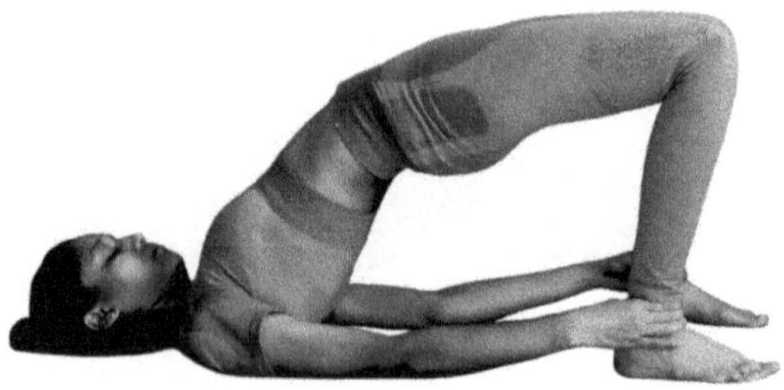

ANANDA BALASANA – Happy Baby Pose

Sanskrit Name: Ānanda Bālāsana - आनन्द बालासन

English Name: Happy Baby Pose

Category of Pose: Supine / Hip Opener / Restorative

Level of Difficulty: Beginner

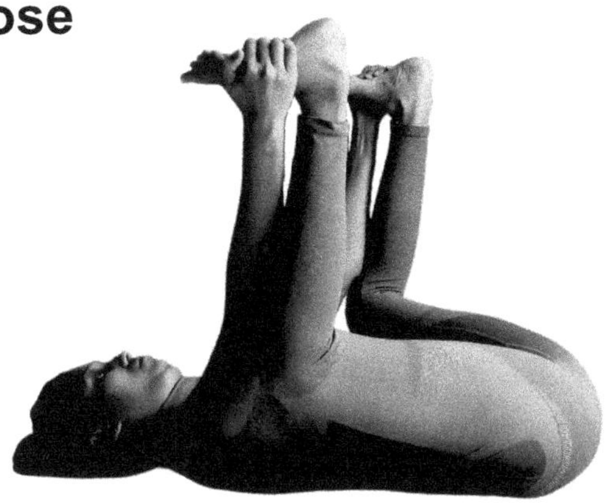

Ananda Balasana

Step-by-Step Instructions:

- Lie flat on your back with knees bent.
- Draw your knees toward your armpits, keeping feet flexed.
- Reach up and hold the outer edges of your feet with your hands (alternatively, hold your ankles or use a strap).
- Ensure your ankles are directly above your knees, forming a 90° angle.
- Gently press your feet down while resisting with your hands, creating gentle traction in the hips.
- Keep the tailbone rooted to the floor, spine neutral, and shoulders relaxed.
- Breathe deeply and hold the pose for 30 seconds to 1 minute.

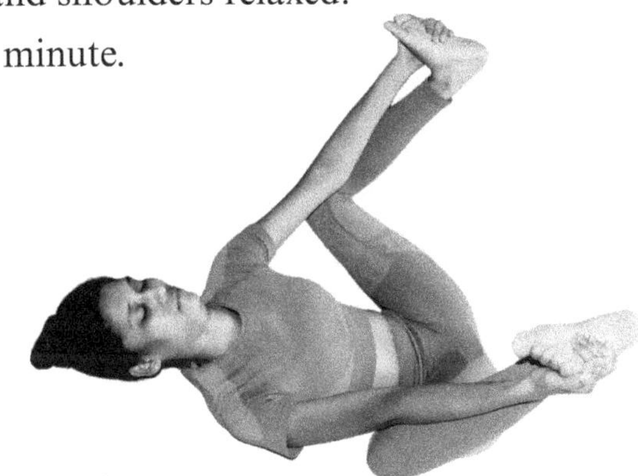

Benefits:

- Deeply opens the hips, groin, and inner thighs.
- Gently stretch the spine and lower back.
- Calms the mind and helps relieve stress and fatigue.
- Aids in digestive health and releases pelvic tension.

Contraindications:

- Knee or hip injuries
- Neck or shoulder issues

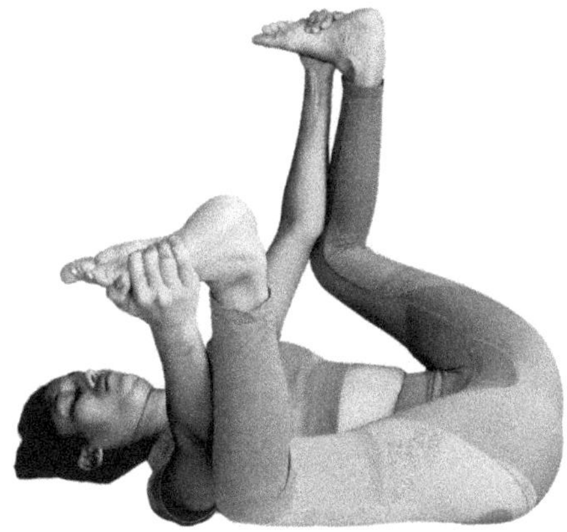

Modifications:

- Use a yoga strap around the soles of the feet for limited reach.
- Place a folded blanket under the head or hips for spinal support.
- Gently rock side to side for a soothing massage effect on the back.

JATHARA PARIVARTANASANA – Supine Spinal Twist

Sanskrit Name: Jathara Parivartānāsana - जठर परिवर्तनासन

English Name: Supine Spinal Twist

Category of Pose: Supine / Twist

Level of Difficulty: Beginner

Step-by-Step Instructions:

- Lie on your back with your arms extended out to the sides in a T-shape, palms facing up.
- Bend your knees and draw them in toward your chest.
- On an exhale, slowly drop both knees to the right, keeping both knees and feet together, and the shoulders grounded.
- Gaze toward your left hand or straight up, whichever is more comfortable for your neck.
- Relax the belly and breathe deeply, holding for 30 seconds to 1 minute.
- Inhale to return the knees to center and repeat on the opposite side.

Benefits:

- Improves spinal mobility and flexibility.
- Releases tension in the spine and lower back.
- Calms the nervous system and helps reduce stress.
- Stimulates the digestive organs and supports detoxification.

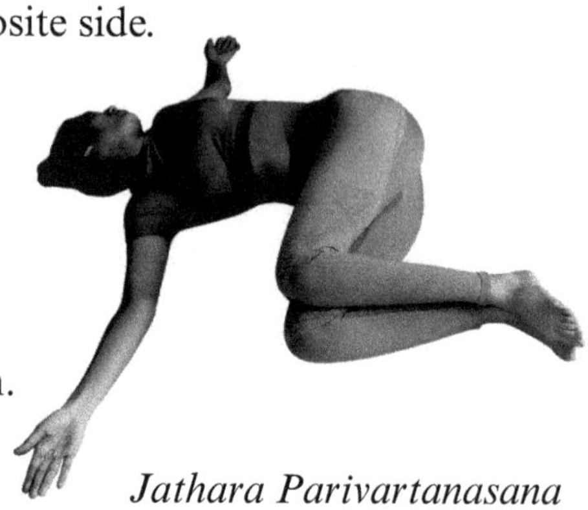

Jathara Parivartanasana

Contraindications:

- Recent spinal, abdominal, or hip surgeries – practice with caution.
- Avoid forcing the knees down if there is lower back pain.

Modifications:

- Place a block between the knees for balanced alignment.
- Keep one leg extended and only twist the top leg across for a gentler variation.

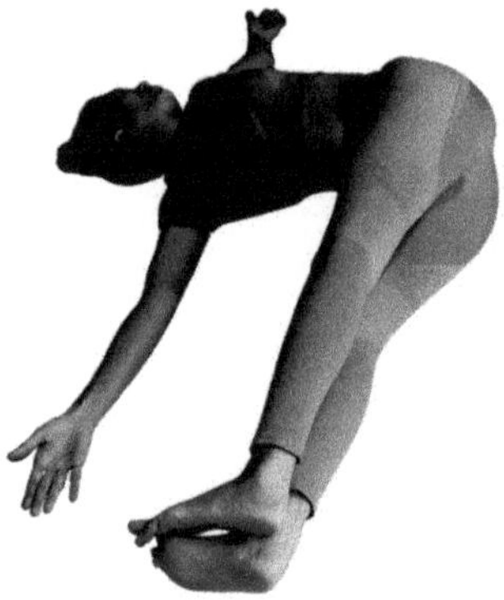

Jathara Parivartanasana V2

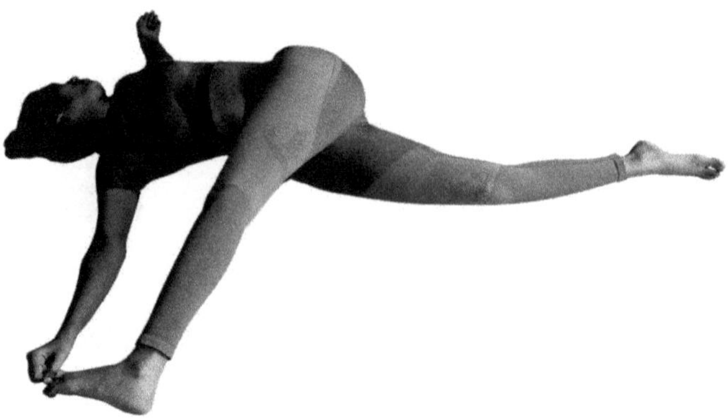

Jathara Parivartanasana V3

MATSYASANA – Fish Pose

Sanskrit Name: Matsyāsana - मत्स्यासन

English Name: Fish Pose

Category of Pose: Supine / Backbend

Level of Difficulty: Beginner to Intermediate

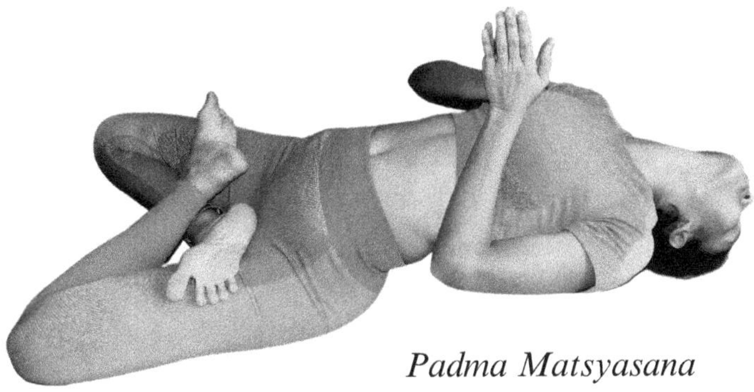

Padma Matsyasana

Step-by-Step Instructions:

- Lie flat on your back with your legs extended and arms by your sides.
- Slide your hands under your buttocks, palms facing down. Bring the elbows closer under your body.
- Inhale, press into your forearms, and lift the chest upward, arching the back.
- Drop the crown of your head gently to the floor, creating a gentle arch in the upper spine.
- Keep legs active and together or in **Padmasana** (Lotus Legs) if **advanced**.
- Breathe deeply and hold for 15–30 seconds, gradually increasing with practice.
- To release, press into your elbows again, gently lift the head, lower the chest, and relax.

Benefits:

- Expands the chest and lungs, improving respiratory function.
- Stimulates the thyroid and parathyroid glands.
- Relieves tension in the neck, shoulders, and upper back.
- Counters the effects of prolonged forward bending or hunching.

Contraindications:

- Severe neck or back injuries – avoid or modify with props.
- Avoid if experiencing dizziness, high blood pressure, or migraines.

Modifications:

- Use a yoga block or bolster under the upper back for a supported version.
- Beginners can keep knees bent with feet flat on the floor.

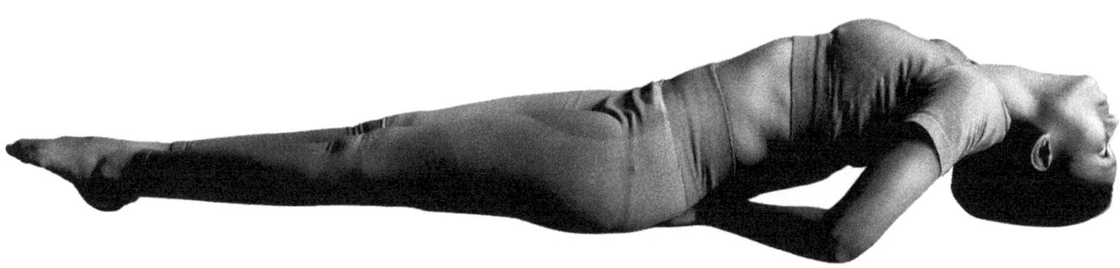

Matsyasana

Prone Yoga Asanas - Belly-Down Poses

MAKARASANA – Crocodile Pose

Sanskrit Name: Makarāsana - मकरासन

English Name: Crocodile Pose

Category of Pose: Prone / Restorative / Meditative

Level of Difficulty: Beginner

Step-by-Step Instructions:

- Lie flat on your stomach, legs extended hip-width apart, toes pointing outward.
- Bend both arms at the elbows and place one palm over the other, then rest your forehead on your hands.
- Keep the chest and shoulders relaxed, allowing your entire body to soften into the mat.
- Close the eyes and breathe deeply into the abdomen, maintaining the position for 1–5 minutes as a rest pose or for longer in relaxation practices.

Benefits:

- Relieves strain from the lower back and relaxes spinal muscles.
- Promotes deep diaphragmatic breathing, calming the nervous system.
- Beneficial for those with scoliosis or slipped disc.
- Gently stimulates digestion by pressing the abdominal area.

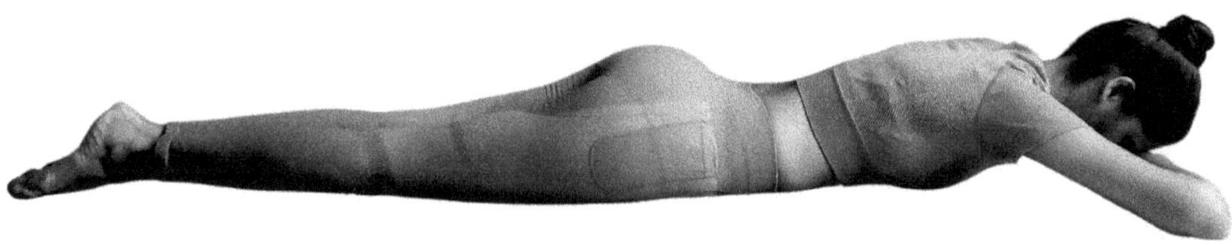

Makarasana

Contraindications:

- Avoid in case of **serious neck or shoulder issues**.

Modifications:

- Place a thin folded blanket under the chest or forehead for extra comfort.
- If shoulder tension arises, extend the arms forward and rest the head to one side.

BHUJANGASANA – Cobra Pose

Sanskrit Name: Bhujangāsana - भुजंगासन
English Name: Cobra Pose
Category of Pose: Prone / Backbend
Level of Difficulty: Beginner

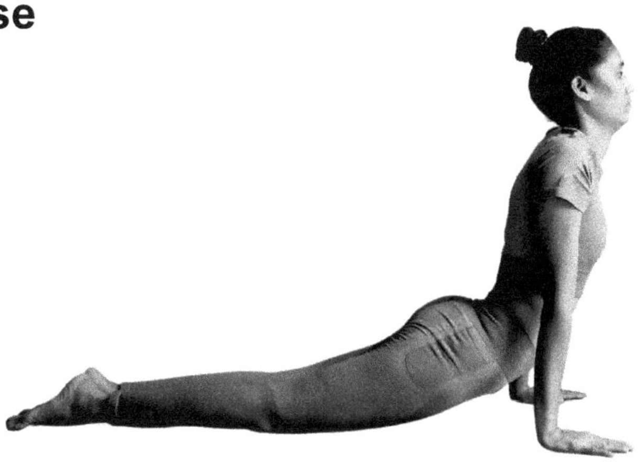

Bhujangasana

Step-by-Step Instructions:

- Lie flat on your stomach, legs extended back with feet hip-width apart, tops of the feet pressing into the mat.
- Place your hands beneath your shoulders, elbows bent and close to the ribcage.
- Inhale, press into your palms, and lift your chest off the floor, engaging the back muscles more than the arms.
- Keep shoulders relaxed, away from the ears, and elbows slightly bent.
- Gaze forward or slightly upward without compressing the neck.
- Hold the pose for 15–30 seconds, breathing steadily.
- To release, exhale, and gently lower your chest and forehead back to the mat.

Benefits:

- Strengthens the spine, shoulders, and arms.
- Opens the chest and lungs, enhancing respiratory capacity.
- Stimulates the abdominal organs, aiding digestion.
- Improves posture and reduces back stiffness.
- Relieves symptoms of fatigue and mild depression.

Contraindications:

- Avoid with severe back injuries, recent abdominal surgeries.
- Not recommended for individuals with carpal tunnel syndrome or hernia.

Modifications:

- For a gentler version, keep elbows on the floor in Sphinx Pose.
- Beginners may raise the chest only slightly while focusing on lengthening the spine.

SALAMBA BHUJANGASANA – Sphinx Pose

Sanskrit Name: Sālamba Bhujangāsana - सलम्ब भुजंगासन

English Name: Supported Cobra / Sphinx Pose

Category of Pose: Prone / Gentle Backbend / Restorative

Level of Difficulty: Beginner

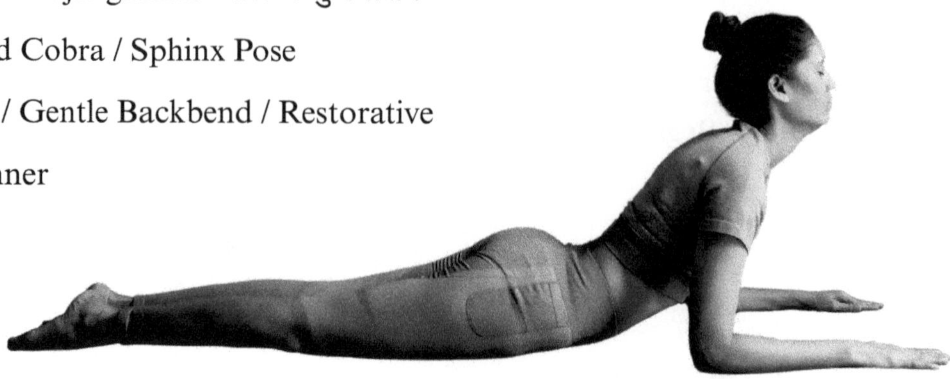

Salamba Bhujangasana

Step-by-Step Instructions:

- Lie flat on your stomach, legs extended back and feet hip-width apart.
- Bring your elbows under your shoulders, forearms parallel on the floor, palms facing down.
- Spread your fingers gently and press the forearms and tops of feet into the mat.
- Inhale, lift the chest and head, lengthening the spine upward without compressing the lower back.
- Keep shoulders relaxed, gaze straight ahead or slightly upward.
- Breathe slowly and remain in the pose for 30 seconds to 2 minutes, depending on comfort.

Benefits:

- Strengthens the spine and muscles of the lower back.
- Promotes gentle spinal extension without straining.
- Stimulates abdominal organs, aiding digestion.
- Opens the heart and chest - improving posture and breath capacity.
- A great preparatory pose for deeper backbends like Bhujangasana.

Contraindications:

- Avoid with severe back injuries, recent abdominal surgeries.

Modifications:

- Place a folded blanket under the pelvis or arms for extra comfort.
- To reduce pressure on the lower back, widen the legs slightly apart.

SALABHASANA – Locust Pose

Sanskrit Name: Śalabhāsana - शलभासन

English Name: Locust Pose

Category of Pose: Prone / Backbend

Level of Difficulty: Beginner to Intermediate

Step-by-Step Instructions:

- Lie face down on your mat, arms alongside the body, palms facing down or tucked under thighs for support.
- Keep the legs together or hip-width apart, tops of the feet pressing into the mat.
- On an inhale, engage the core and glutes, then lift the head, chest, arms, and legs off the ground.
- Keep the arms straight and extended back, palms facing down or in toward the body.
- Gaze slightly forward or down to keep the neck neutral.
- Breathe steadily and hold the pose for 20–30 seconds, or 3–5 breaths.
- Exhale to lower down gently, turning the head to one side to rest.

Benefits:

- Strengthens the back, glutes, hamstrings, and shoulders.
- Improves posture and helps relieve lower back pain.
- Stimulates digestive organs, promoting better digestion.
- Encourages lung expansion and deeper breathing.
- Boosts mental focus and energy.

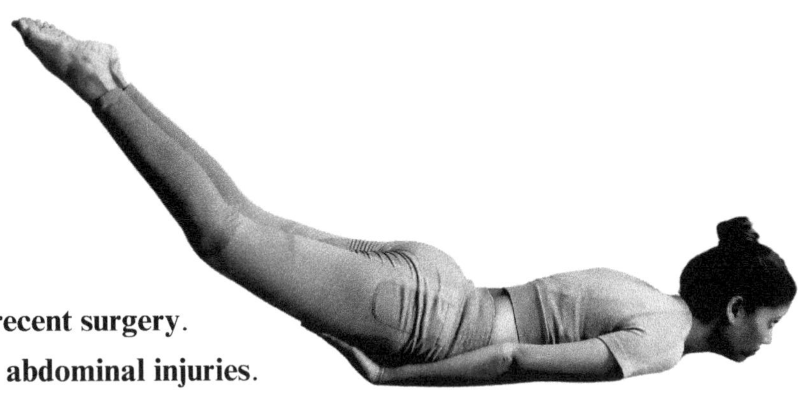

Salabhasana

Contraindications:

- Use caution in case of **hernia or recent surgery**.
- Avoid with **serious back, neck, or abdominal injuries**.

Modifications:

- Keep hands under thighs for more support.
- Use a folded blanket under the pelvis for comfort.
- Lift just the lower body if the full lift is too intense.

ARDHA SHALABHASANA – Half Locust Pose

Sanskrit Name: Ardha Śalabhāsana - अर्ध शलभासन
English Name: Half Locust Pose
Category of Pose: Prone / Backbend
Level of Difficulty: Beginner

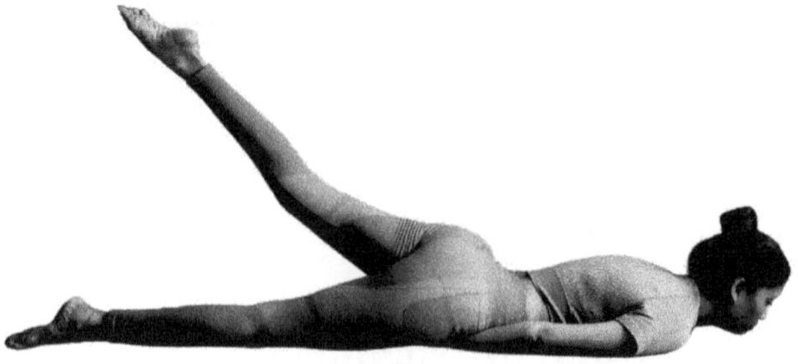

Ardha Salabhasana

Step-by-Step Instructions:

- Lie face down on your mat, arms alongside the body, palms facing upward or tucked under thighs for support.
- Keep legs together, chin or forehead resting gently on the floor.
- On an inhale, engage the glutes and lift the right leg (straight and active) off the floor as high as comfortable without rotating the hip.
- Keep the pelvis grounded and shoulders relaxed.
- Breathe normally and hold the position for 3–5 breaths.
- Exhale to lower the leg, rest briefly, then repeat on the left side.
- Optional: Repeat each side 2–3 times, alternating legs.

Benefits:

- Strengthens lower back, glutes, and hamstrings.
- Prepares the body for full Salabhasana (Locust Pose).
- Gently stimulates abdominal organs, aiding digestion.
- Enhances body awareness and spinal alignment.

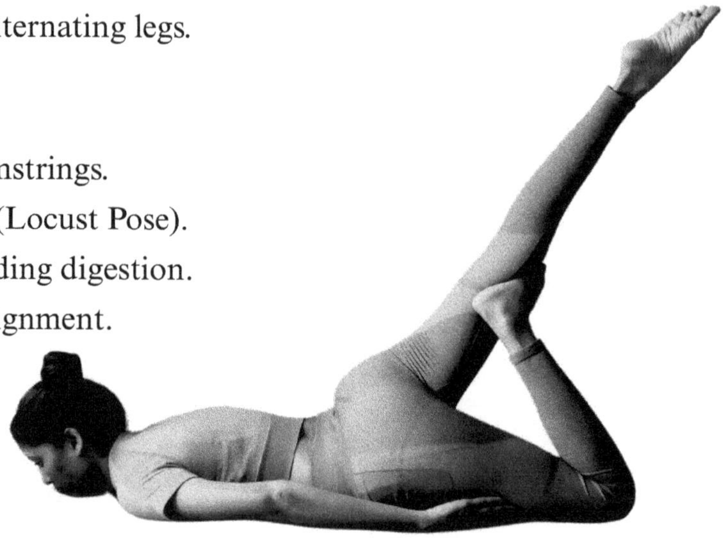

Ardha Salabhasana

Contraindications:

- Avoid with lower back pain, herniated disc, or abdominal surgery.
- Practice mindfully if dealing with sciatica or hip issues.

Modifications:

- Use a folded blanket under the pelvis for added support.
- Reduce lift height if there's discomfort in the back or hips.
- Beginners can place a thin cushion under the ankle for ease.

DHANURASANA – Bow Pose

Sanskrit Name: Dhanurāsana - धनुरासन
English Name: Bow Pose
Category of Pose: Prone / Backbend
Level of Difficulty: Intermediate

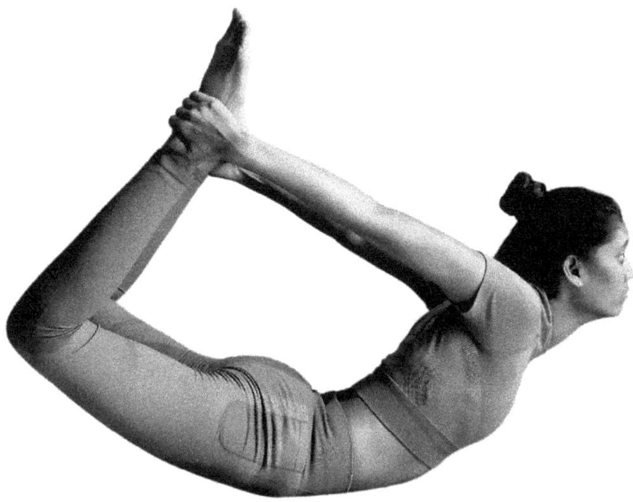

Dhanurasana

Step-by-Step Instructions:

- Lie face down on the mat with arms by your sides and chin resting on the floor.
- Bend both knees and bring the heels toward the buttocks.
- Reach back with both hands and grasp the ankles (not the tops of the feet).
- On an inhale, lift the chest and thighs off the floor simultaneously, creating a bow shape with the body.
- Pull the ankles away from the back, using the legs to help lift the upper body, keeping the knees hip-width apart.
- Gaze forward or slightly upward, keeping breath steady and abdominal muscles engaged.
- Hold for 3–5 breaths, then gently release on an exhale, returning to the starting position.

Benefits:

- Strengthens the back, glutes, hamstrings, and shoulders.
- Improves spinal flexibility and posture.
- Stimulates digestive and reproductive organs.
- Opens the chest and lungs, enhancing breathing capacity.

Contraindications:

- Avoid in case of hernia, abdominal surgery, neck issues, or spinal injuries.

Modifications:

- Use a yoga strap looped around the ankles if reaching them is challenging.
- Keep the thighs lower for beginners to reduce pressure on the spine.
- Place a blanket under the hips for more comfort and support.

MARJARĪĀSANA & BITILĀSANA – Cat-Cow Pose

Sanskrit Names:

- **Marjariasana** - मर्जरीआसन – Cat Pose
- **Bitilasana** - बितिलासन – Cow Pose

English Names: Cat Pose & Cow Pose

Category of Pose: Kneeling / Spinal Mobility

Level of Difficulty: Beginner

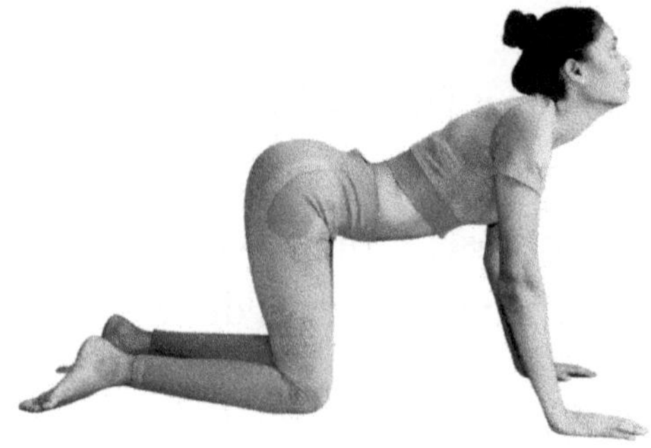

Bitilasana - Cow Pose

Step-by-Step Instructions:

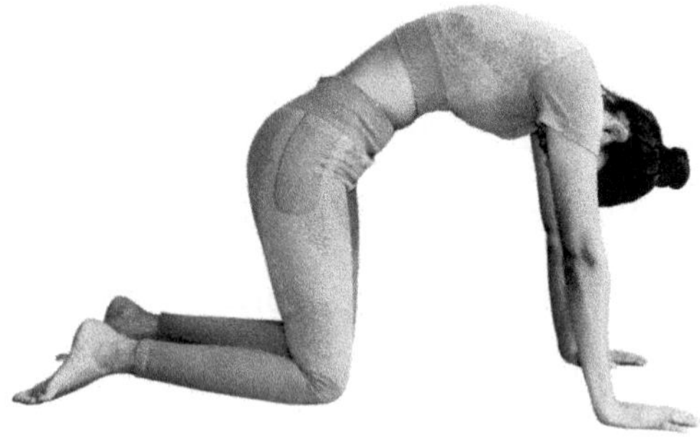

Marjariasana - Cat Pose

1. Begin on all **fours** in a tabletop position:

- Wrists under shoulders
- Knees under hips
- Spine in a neutral position, gaze down
- Fingers spread wide, pressing evenly into the palms

2. Bitilasana (Cow Pose):

- Inhale: Drop the belly, lift the chest and tailbone upward
- Gaze slightly upward (avoid compressing the neck)
- Open the front body and arch the spine gently

3. Marjariasana (Cat Pose):

- Exhale: Round the spine, tuck the tailbone and draw the chin toward the chest
- Press into the hands and broaden the upper back
- Engage the core and stretch the back body

4. Continue to flow with the breath, alternating between the two poses for 5–10 rounds.

Benefits:

- Improves spinal mobility and flexibility
- Gently stretches the back, neck, and abdomen
- Warms up the body before deeper asanas
- Encourages mindful breathing and body awareness
- Helps relieve tension from the back and shoulders
- Stimulates the digestive organs

Contraindications:

- Avoid or modify with **wrist or knee injuries**
- Use caution in case of **neck pain** - keep the gaze neutral

Modifications:

- Use a **blanket under the knees** for support
- If wrist discomfort occurs, make fists or use a **Block**
- Practice the movement **seated** or standing if kneeling isn't accessible

Counter Pose:

- Rest in **Balasana (Child's Pose)** after the sequence to neutralize the spine.

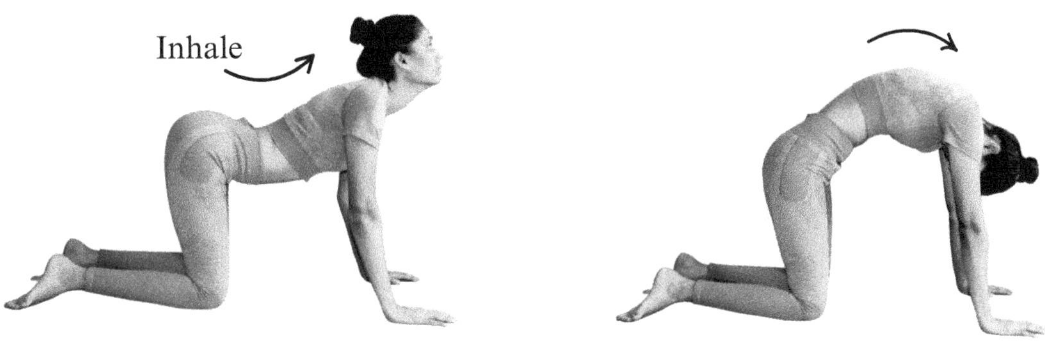

Performing Cat -Cow Pose

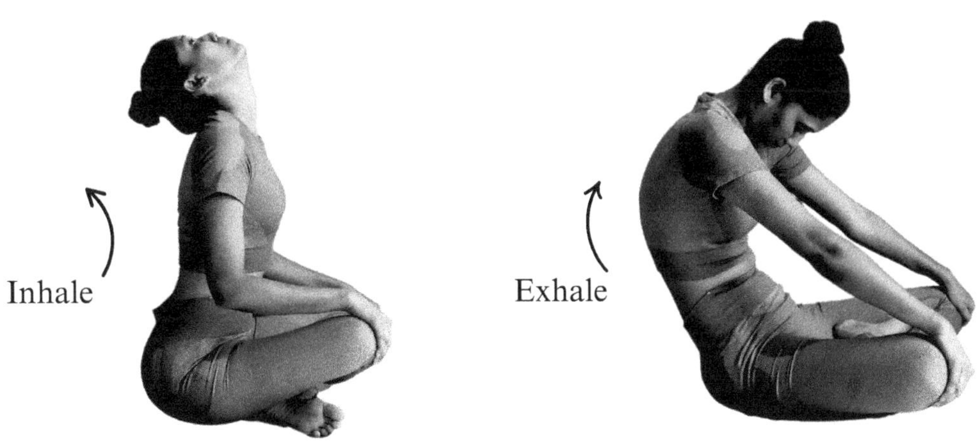

Performing Seated Cat -Cow Pose

PHALAKĀSANA – Plank Pose

Sanskrit Name: Phalakasana - फलकासन

English Name: Plank Pose

Category of Pose: Arm Balance / Core Strengthening

Level of Difficulty: Beginner to Intermediate

Step-by-Step Instructions:

- Begin in Tabletop position (hands and knees on the mat).
- Step both feet back, one at a time, straightening the legs behind you.
- Align shoulders directly over wrists, and spread fingers wide for a firm foundation.
- Engage the core, keeping the body in a straight line from head to heels.
- Keep the neck neutral, gaze down slightly ahead of the fingers.
- Hold the pose for 30 seconds to 1 minute, breathing steadily.
- To release, lower the knees or transition to Balasana or Makarasana.

Benefits:

- Strengthens the arms, shoulders, wrists, and core
- Builds stamina and endurance
- Prepares the body for arm balances and advanced poses
- Improves posture and spinal alignment
- Activates deep stabilizing muscles

Contraindications:

- Wrist or shoulder injuries
- High blood pressure – avoid long holds

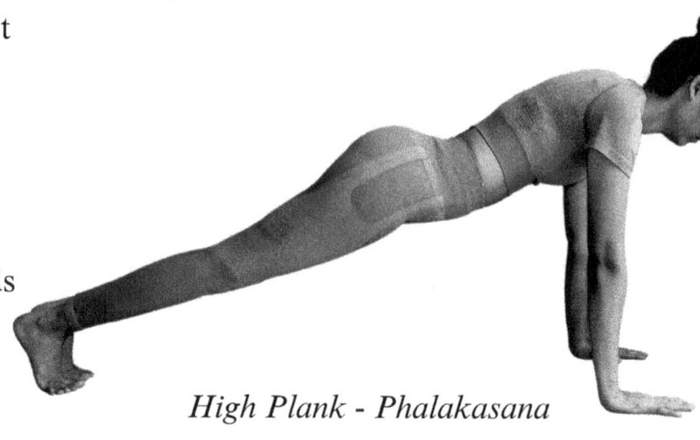

High Plank - Phalakasana

Modifications:

- Drop knees to the mat for a modified Plank
- Use a folded mat or blanket under the wrists if needed

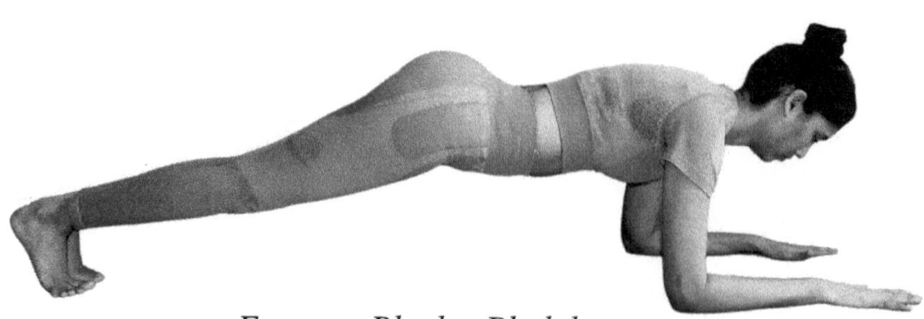

Forearm Plank - Phalakasana

Inverted Yoga Asanas - Upside-Down Poses

SARVANGĀSANA – Shoulder Stand Pose

Sanskrit Name: Sarvangasana - सर्वांगासन

English Name: Shoulder Stand

Category of Pose: Inversion

Level of Difficulty: Intermediate to Advanced

Step-by-Step Instructions:

- Begin lying flat on your back with arms by your sides, palms down.
- On an inhale, lift both legs up to 90 degrees.
- Press your palms into the mat and lift the hips off the floor, supporting your lower back with your hands.
- Walk your elbows in closer and ensure the upper arms are firm on the mat.
- Gently extend the legs upward, aiming to stack hips, torso, and legs in one straight line over the shoulders.
- Keep your neck relaxed and eyes looking upward. Do not turn the head.
- Hold the pose for 30 seconds to 2 minutes, breathing evenly.
- To come out, bend the knees, and slowly lower the spine down to the mat.

Benefits:

- Stimulates the thyroid and parathyroid glands
- Enhances blood circulation to the brain and upper body
- Calms the nervous system, reduces stress and fatigue
- Improves digestion and supports lymphatic drainage
- Strengthens shoulders, core, and legs

Contraindications:

- Neck injuries or cervical spondylitis
- High blood pressure or heart conditions, menstruation

Modifications:

- Practice **with wall support** for balance
- Use **folded blankets under the shoulders** to reduce neck compression

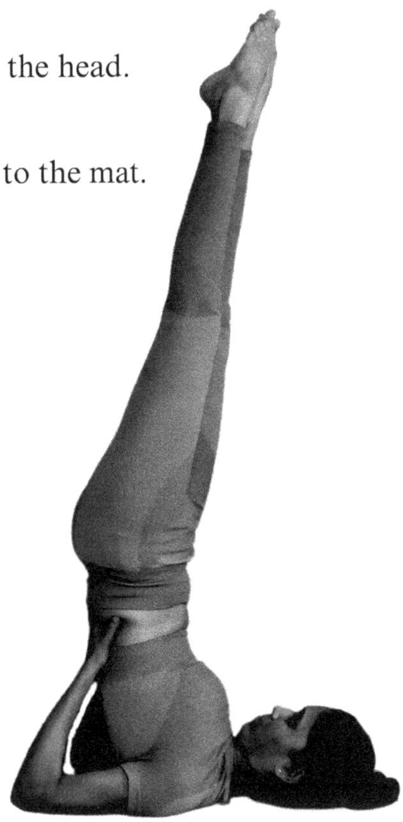

Sarvangasana

Counter Pose: Matsyasana - Fish Pose

HALĀSANA – Plow Pose

Sanskrit Name: Halasana - हलासन

English Name: Plow Pose

Category of Pose: Inversion

Level of Difficulty: Intermediate

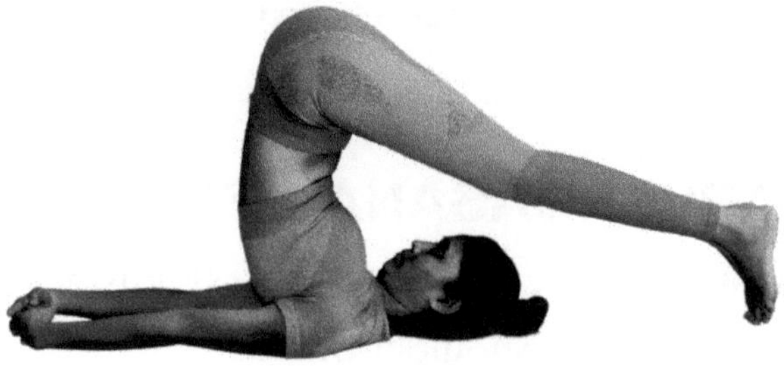

Halasana

Step-by-Step Instructions:

- Begin lying flat on your back, arms alongside the body, palms facing down.
- Inhale and raise your legs to 90 degrees, then press into the arms to lift the hips off the mat.
- Support the lower back with your hands as you roll the legs overhead.
- Gently lower the toes towards the floor behind the head, keeping the legs straight.
- Once the toes touch (or come close), release the hands and extend the arms flat on the mat, palms down.
- Keep the neck long, gaze upward, and do not turn the head.
- Breathe steadily and hold for 15 seconds to 1 minute, depending on your level.

Benefits:

- Deeply stretches the spine, shoulders, and hamstrings
- Calms the brain and nervous system, relieves stress and fatigue
- Stimulates the thyroid gland and improves metabolism
- Aids digestion and promotes healthy abdominal organs
- Improves flexibility and spinal mobility

Contraindications:

- Neck injuries or cervical issues
- High blood pressure, glaucoma, or inner ear disorders, menstruation
- Recent abdominal surgery or hernia, or menstruation

Modifications:

- Place a folded blanket under the shoulders to reduce neck strain
- If toes don't reach the floor, rest them on a chair or block
- Bend the knees slightly for tight hamstrings or lower back sensitivity
- Beginners may keep hands on the lower back for support

Counter Pose: Matsyasana - Fish Pose

CHAKRĀSANA – Wheel Pose

Sanskrit Name: Chakrāsana - चक्रासन

English Name: Wheel Pose

Category of Pose: Backbend / Inversion

Level of Difficulty: Intermediate to Advanced

Step-by-Step Instructions:

- Lie flat on your back, bend your knees and place the feet hip-width apart, close to the buttocks.
- Bend your elbows and place your palms on the floor beside your head, fingers pointing toward the shoulders.
- Inhale, press into your hands and feet, lifting the hips and chest upward.
- Straighten your arms and legs as much as possible, bringing your body into a full arch, resembling a wheel.
- Keep your neck relaxed, head hanging gently.
- Breathe deeply and hold for 5–15 seconds initially, gradually increasing with practice.

Benefits:

- Deeply strengthens the arms, legs, spine, and shoulders
- Expands the chest and lungs, improving respiratory function
- Stimulates the thyroid, pituitary glands, and nervous system
- Boosts energy levels and combats fatigue and depression
- Enhances the flexibility of the spine and hip joints

Contraindications:

- Wrist, shoulder, or back injuries
- Menstruation, Heart conditions, or high BP
- Recent surgery (especially abdominal or spinal)

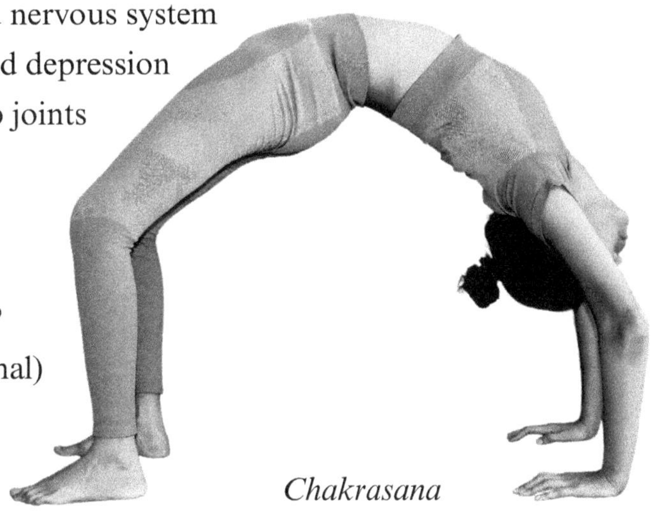

Chakrasana

Modifications:

- Use a yoga wheel or place hands on blocks to reduce wrist strain
- Practice Bridge Pose (Setu Bandhasana) as a preparatory alternative
- Ask the teacher or partner to support your lower back during lift.

Counter Poses: Paschimottanasana, Balasana.

Chapter 4: Asana Modifications

Why Modify Asanas?

Every student arrives on the mat with a unique body, history, and intention. Asana modifications are intentional adjustments made to yoga:

- **Safe** for those with injuries or mobility issues
- **Accessible** to all body types and age groups
- A tool for building **confidence and consistency**

Use of Props in Yoga

Yoga props are supportive tools that help practitioners experience the benefits of a pose with **greater ease, stability, injury prevention, and alignment**. They allow both beginners and advanced students to explore poses safely and mindfully.

Common Yoga Props & Their Uses

Prop	Purpose & Benefits
Yoga Block	Brings the floor closer in standing or seated poses, supports hips, hands, or back.
Yoga Strap	Helps in reaching feet or hands in forward folds and binds, improves range of motion.
Yoga Wheel	Helps in enhancing flexibility, improve balance and deepen stretches in yoga practice
Yoga Blanket	Provides cushioning for knees, spine, or head; aids in seated and restorative postures.
Bolster	Offers full-body support in restorative and seated poses, promotes deep relaxation.
Wall	Enhances balance, alignment, and support in inversions and standing postures.
Chair	Assists in therapeutic or accessible yoga, supports deeper explorations of postures.
Eye Pillow	Used during final relaxation to encourage stillness and soothe the nervous system.

Common Modification Strategies

Modification Type	Description
Use of Props	Blocks, straps, bolsters, blankets, chairs, or walls to support the body
Range Adjustment	Reducing depth, angle, or stretch in the pose
Alignment Adjustments	Altering foot, hand, or hip placement for safety or comfort
Postural Variations	Switching to a similar but less intense or more accessible version
Supportive Entry/Exit	Adding transitions or steps to enter/exit safely
Chair or Wall Support	Offering seated or supported alternatives for standing/balance poses

Examples of Modifications for Common Asanas

Vrikshasana (Tree Pose)

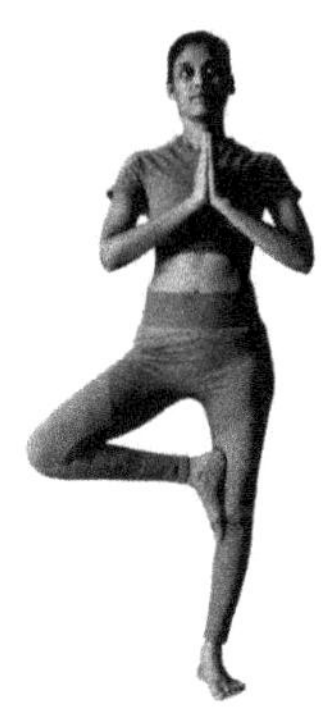

- Place the foot below the knee or on the ankle
- Use a wall for balance support
- Hands in a prayer position instead of overhead

Paschimottanasana - Seated Forward Bend

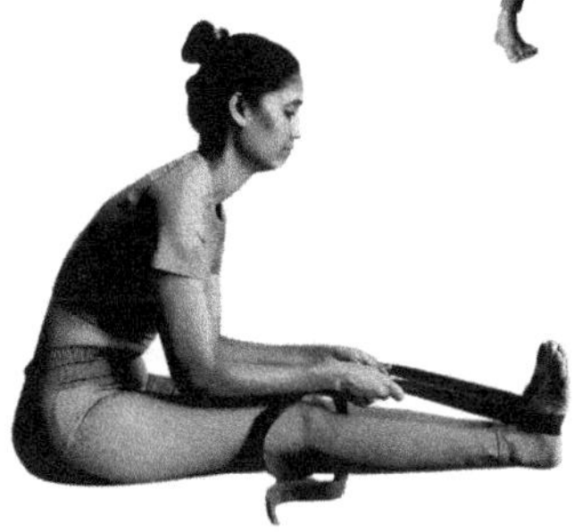

- Sit on a folded blanket to tilt the pelvis forward
- Place a strap around the feet if hands don't reach
- Slightly bend knees for tight hamstrings

Padmasana – Lotus Pose

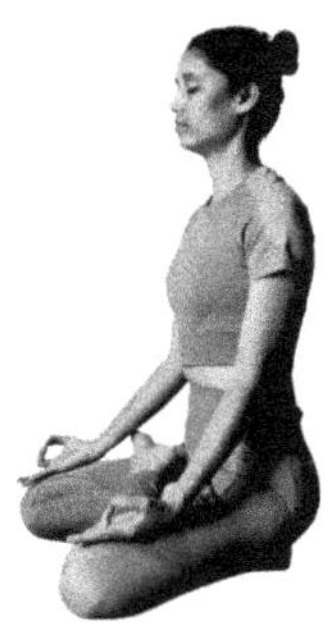

- Elevate the hips by sitting on a folded blanket or block
- Sit in Sukhasana or Ardha Padmasana (Half Lotus)

Language Matters: How to Offer Modifications Gracefully

Avoid saying:

- *"If you can't do the full pose, try this..."*

Instead try:

- "Here's another option that might feel better today."
- "You're still doing the pose - just in a way that honors your body."
- "Choose the variation where you can breathe freely and stay steady."

Teaching Tips

- Introduce props as a **tool, not a crutch**
- Demonstrate both the **classical** and **modified versions**
- Normalize the use of props and adjustments in every class
- Empower students to **self-modify** without feeling like they're falling behind
- Encourage students to check in with their own energy and intention each day

1. Block
2. Strap
3. Wheel
4. Chair
5. Bolster
6. Blanket
7. Eye Pillow

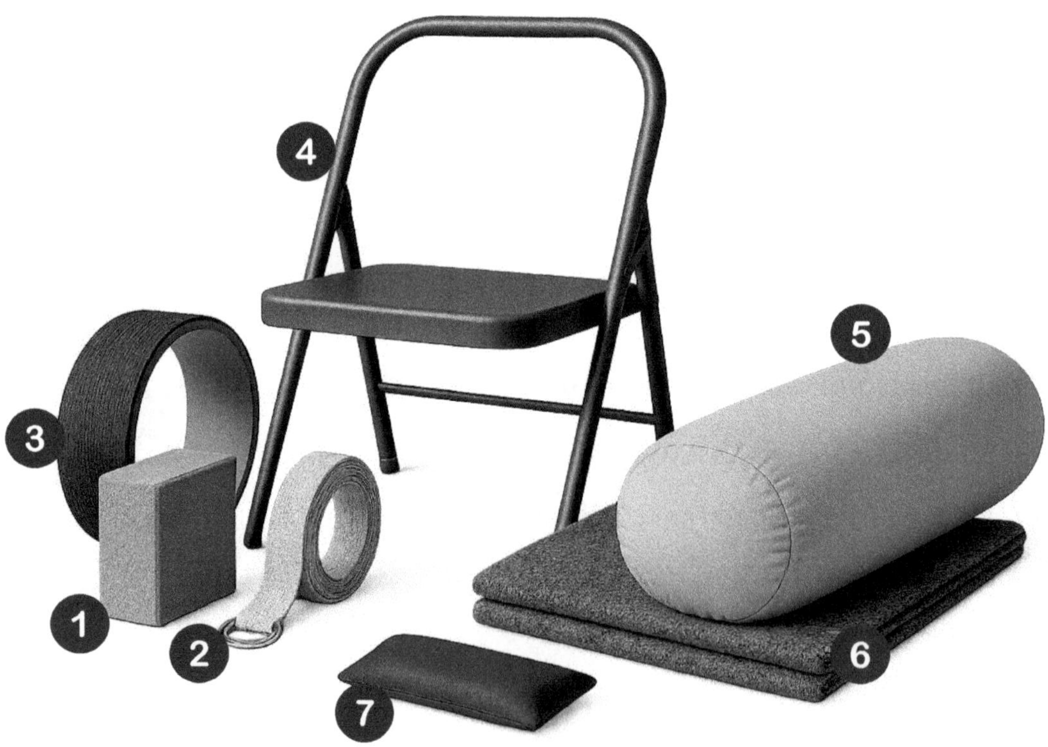

Yoga Props

Chapter 5: Teaching Methodology

Verbal Cues & Hands-On Adjustments

A good teacher communicates not just *what* to do but *how and why*, in a way that's empowering, inclusive, and clear. In yoga, this is done through **verbal cues**, **hands-on adjustments**, and **energetic presence**. As a teacher, learning to **guide students safely and effectively** with both words and touch is essential for transformation, connection, and growth.

Effective Verbal Cueing

Verbal cues are the **primary language of teaching**: They help students move safely, focus inward, and refine their practice without relying on demonstration.

Best Practices for Verbal Cueing:

- **Be Clear:** Use simple, direct language ("Root down through your feet", "Lift your chest gently")
- **Be Concise:** Fewer words = more space for awareness
- **Cue Action, Not Just Shape:** Focus on what the student should do with their body ("Draw the navel in" vs "Engage your core")
- **Cue Breath & Awareness:** "Inhale to lengthen the spine… exhale to fold deeper"
- **Sequence Your Cues:**
    - Foundation (what's grounded)
    - Action (movement or engagement)
    - Direction (where to move or expand)

Types of Verbal Cues:

- **Alignment Cues**: "Stack shoulder over wrist"
- **Energetic Cues**: "Shine the heart forward"
- **Anatomical Cues**: "Hinge at the hips, not the waist"
- **Supportive Cues**: "There's no need to force it, listen to your edge."

Demonstration & Observation

Demonstration & Observation

A great yoga teacher knows **when to demonstrate**, **when to observe**, and how to strike the right balance between **showing and seeing**. Demonstration offers a **visual reference** for students, while observation allows the teacher to **assess alignment, energy, and safety** in the room.

Both are crucial tools in the teacher's toolkit, and learning to switch between them smoothly creates a more **interactive, responsive** teaching experience.

Demonstration

Purpose

To visually convey alignment, movement, transitions, and energy within a posture.

When to Use Demonstration

Demonstration is especially useful when:

- Reinforcing verbal instructions
- Introducing a **new or complex pose**
- Teaching **beginners or visual learners**
- Explaining **transitions or sequencing**
- Illustrating **alignment, modifications, or common mistakes**

Best Practices for Demonstrating

- **Be Clear and Visible**
    - Face your students unless mirroring.
    - Position yourself where the whole class can see.
    - Move slowly and mindfully to emphasize key actions.

- **Mirror When Necessary**
    - Use opposite sides to match students' movement.
    - Example: You step your left foot back so students step their right.

- **Talk Through the Movement**
  - Describe what you're doing clearly.
  - Synchronize cueing with movement.

- **Use Props**
  - Demonstrate with blocks, straps, or walls to encourage support and accessibility.

- **Limit Demonstration**
  - Don't overuse demo; balance it with observation to stay present with students.
  - Avoid demoing during deep or meditative practices like Savasana or Pranayama.

Observation

Observation allows you to:

- See how students are **responding to your cues**
- Identify misalignments or **unhelpful patterns**
- Offer **real-time cues, modifications, and support**
- Read the **energy of the room -** are students anxious, focused, overwhelmed, or disengaged?

What to Observe

- **Alignment** – Are joints stacked and muscles engaged properly?
- **Effort vs. Ease** – Are students straining or flowing smoothly?
- **Breath** – Is the breath fluid and calm or restricted?
- **Facial Expressions** – Do they suggest discomfort, stress, or ease?
- **Energy Levels** – Who might need encouragement or grounding?
- **Use of Props** – Are they using supports effectively or hesitantly?

Observation Strategies in the Classroom

- **Walk the Room:** Observe the students from different angles and stay aware of every corner of the room.
- **Soften Your Gaze:** Use peripheral awareness to spot subtle misalignments or tension.
- **Tune into Energy:** Feel the collective energy of the room, fast, anxious, calm, sleepy?
- **Observe Without Judging:** Be a curious and compassionate witness, not a critic.
- **Match Observation to Cueing:** If you notice common misalignments, address them with inclusive verbal cues.

Chapter 6: Giving and Receiving Feedback

Feedback is one of the most powerful tools for growth and transformation, whether you're offering it to students or receiving it as a teacher-in-training. In yoga, feedback must be delivered with kindness, clarity, and respect, honoring the vulnerability that often comes with both teaching and learning.

Why Feedback Matters in Yoga Teaching

- Helps **refine teaching skills** through reflection
- Encourages **self-awareness and confidence**
- Builds a culture of **support and accountability**
- Allows teachers to better serve diverse student needs

Giving Feedback – How to Offer It Constructively

Giving feedback isn't about criticism, it's about **supporting growth** with honesty and kindness.

Principles of Constructive Feedback

- **Be Timely** - Offer feedback soon after the class/session when it's still fresh.
- **Be Specific** - Instead of saying "That was good," try "Your pacing during Sun Salutations was smooth and well-timed."
- **Balance Positive and Constructive Points**
    - Use the "Sandwich Technique":
        - Start with a strength
        - Gently offer an area for improvement
        - End with encouragement or another strength
- **Focus on Behaviors, Not Personality** - Example: Say "You moved quickly through the warm-up" instead of "You seemed impatient."
- **Offer Suggestions, Not Demands -** "You might consider slowing your cues during transitions to allow students more space."
- **Use "I" Statements** - Own your perspective: "I noticed...," "I felt...," "I appreciated..."
- **Deliver with Compassion** - Let your tone be respectful, calm, and clear; never judgmental.

Receiving Feedback – How to Stay Open & Grounded

Receiving feedback with grace is a sign of inner maturity. It's not always easy, but it's always valuable when approached with the right mindset.

Practices for Receiving Feedback

- **Stay Receptive:** Breathe deeply and remain present while listening.
- **Listen Fully:** Avoid interrupting or defending. Absorb first; reflect later.
- **Reflect, Don't React:** Take time to sit with the feedback before emotionally responding.
- **Ask for Clarity:** If something feels unclear, ask, "Can you explain what you meant by that?"
- **Extract the Truth:** Even if some feedback feels off, see if there's a useful thread you can apply.
- **Say Thank You:** Express gratitude - even if the feedback feels uncomfortable.

Peer Feedback in Teacher Training

During yoga teacher training, peer feedback becomes a valuable tool for collaborative learning. Students grow not only by receiving feedback from trainers but also by **offering it to one another.**

- Establish a **safe, kind, and curious environment**
- Create a respectful circle or group-sharing format.
- Normalize feedback as a gift, not a judgment.
- Frame it as **"We grow together,"** not as competition

Sample Feedback Prompts (For Practice Sessions)

- "One thing I appreciated about your teaching was…"
- "One suggestion I have for you is…"
- "You held space beautifully when…"
- "Consider experimenting with…"

Conclusion & Reflection

As you complete this journey through postural practice, remember that asanas are not endpoints—they are invitations. Every yoga pose is a doorway to inner awareness, a mirror reflecting where you are, what you feel, and how deeply you are present.

Mastery of asanas isn't about touching your toes or balancing on your hands. It's about how skillfully, humbly, and compassionately you guide yourself and others into alignment with the moment.

In your own teaching, focus not on the aesthetics of the pose, but on the experience it creates—a balance between effort and ease, breath and body, structure and spirit.

Teach asana with the awareness of function, the clarity of intention, and the humility of a student—always learning, always listening.

Final Reflection Prompts:

- Which category of postures do I feel most connected to—and why?
- How do I define alignment in my own body today?
- What adjustments or modifications do I want to explore more deeply?
- Why is "Receiving and Giving Feedback" important?

Wish You Health. Peace. Harmony

In gratitude,

Raushan Yoganta
Founder & CEO, Yoganta

www.ingramcontent.com/pod-product-compliance
Ingram Content Group UK Ltd.
Pitfield, Milton Keynes, MK11 3LW, UK
UKHW061540190726
13845UKWH00031B/1133

9 789334 309690